THE WINSTON STORY

The tale of a dog and his family; His epic battle with cancer and their courageous faith to see him through.

Written by
Tim A. Rupard

Published by
Good Dog Reads Publishing

A division of RAR Enterprises
Auburn, GA

COPYRIGHT

Published By: Good Dog Reads Publishing
A Division of RAR Enterprises
P.O. Box 133 Auburn, GA 3011

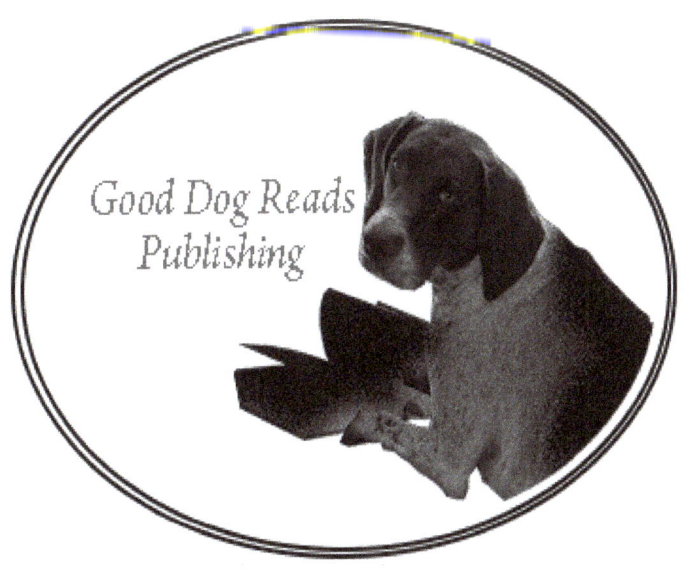

1 Peter 5:6-7

6. Therefore humble yourselves under the mighty hand of God, that He may exalt you in due time,

7. casting all your care upon Him, for He cares for you.

TABLE OF CONTENTS

DEDICATED TO
MURRAY DEWITT WOODWARD

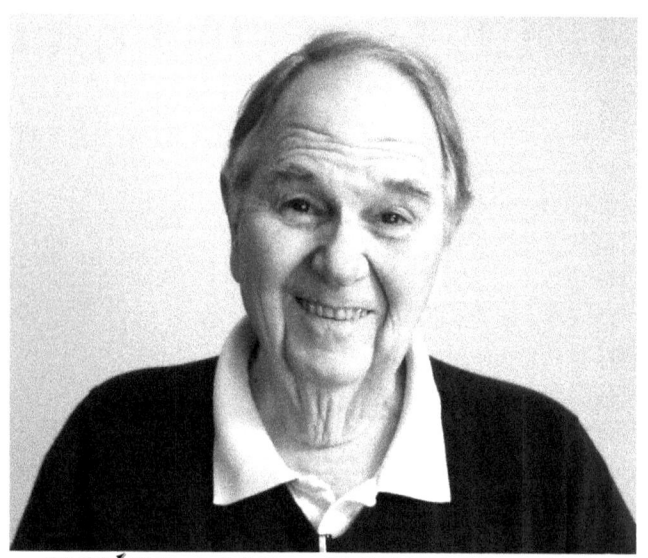

MAY 30, 1942 - MARCH 20, 2020

To my dear friend Dewitt,

You were told, by our Father, to tell me to "Write the Story" before you ever knew there was a story. You had no idea what you would begin in my life, nor how our brief encounter would change the lives of my family, friends, and maybe many others. You were simply doing what you always seemed to be doing; Going about your Father's business.

Thank you, brother.

It grieves me so that you were unable to read the finished edition, but I feel your spirit when I sit to write this, I hope and believe you are rejoicing with every key stroke, as we near the end of this journey. Go rest high upon that mountain, my friend.

FOREWORD

BY
Travis Rutland

I am so honored and pleased that Tim Rupard asked me to write this foreword. He is my dear friend and it has been awesome to see him spiritually grow and mature over the years. I am excited about this book and what it will do in the lives of many people.

In Mark 6, Jesus returns to His hometown of Nazareth. The people listen to Him teach and then ask, "Is this not the son of Mary? Is this not the brother of James?" They know Jesus but they refuse to believe in Jesus. Then, the Bible gives us an astonishing verse. It says in Mark 6:5, "And Jesus could do no mighty works there." This verse begs the question of why. Why could Jesus do no mighty works? Is unbelief Jesus' kryptonite? Was the doubt of the people of Nazareth more powerful than the miraculous power of Jesus? Absolutely not! The reason Jesus did no mighty works there was because no one asked Him. They refused to ask the Messiah to raise the dead or heal the blind. Jesus had the power. However, the people did not believe in Jesus. So, they did not ask Him.

I have known and been close friends with Tim for almost 6 years. The story you will read is about a regular man, his regular family, and their regular dog. Everyone in this story, myself included, are very ordinary. This is not a story about extraordinary people. It is instead simply a story about people who were willing to ask God. People who were willing to pray. People who were willing to believe. People who were willing to fast and fall down on their faces before God and cry out to Him. The point of this story is not that anyone in it is amazing. This story is about ordinary people calling out to an extraordinary God.

Jesus returning to Nazareth is an example of missed opportunities. People who had access to the power of God and absolutely would not ask for a miracle. My hope is that this story of Tim and Winston will encourage you to pray big prayers. We all have problems. We all have difficulties in our life that require supernatural intervention. God wants us to ask Him and He wants to intervene in those issues. As Paul tells us in Ephesians 3:20, "God is able to do exceedingly abundantly above all that we ask or think."

My prayer is that this simple story of healing and miracles will birth something new inside of every single reader. James 4:2 tells us, "You do not have because you do not ask." Allow this story to inspire you. Pray big prayers! Believe in big miracles! We serve a big, big God!

Pastor Travis Rutland

PREFACE

ONLY THE GOOD DIE YOUNG, OR NOT

Life. Despite how long and painful it can be, it is the thing that most of us wish we could extend and increase. When we were young we wanted to be older, never really considering the associated hazards. We didn't fear sickness or disease, we never thought about suffering with cancer or dementia, we weren't worried about high blood pressure or aging eyes. Most of us didn't even know what the term colonoscopy meant, nor did we care. Those things were too far in the future to be of concern. We just lived. When I was twenty, I thought fifty was so far away. Now I am fifty-one and seventy feels way too close! I always thought, "If I live to eighty, I'll be happy!" Nope… I want to live to a hundred if I can have my loved ones with me until then! I used to go hard from before sun up to way past sundown. Now, I groan to get off the couch. If I work hard for one day I pay for it for three. When I was young

I would have jumped off a ten foot wall to the pavement and ran down the street... now, I find I will go a long way around to keep from jumping 3 feet and if I run down the street, it would be because something very scary is chasing me and I've run out of bullets! Now, people I knew when I was much younger are dying as old men and women and their diseases scare me. I used to hear the old people say, as you get older the years just go by faster. I would just nod my head and smile at those comments. Now, I know. They DO! They go by faster! At this rate, by the time I'm seventy, a year will feel like a month and I won't be able to remember longer than a minute at the time!

It seems backwards. It seems like it should slow down as you get older for some reason. But it doesn't. Folks say, "Time flies when you're having fun." Well, I had a lot more fun when I was a kid. I didn't worry about bills or kids or deadlines or any other responsibilities. Fun was an everyday part of life. I still have fun but not like I did then. So if time flies when you're having fun then shouldn't it slow down when you're not having as much fun? Yet, it seems to speed up every year, regardless of the amounts of fun I am having. This getting older thing is not fun!

Sickness seems to be all around me. People that I have known for decades are gone. More often than ever, I hear people who are dear to me have contracted some sort of life-altering illness and often I think to myself, "That hardly seems right or fair, they are such good people, they don't deserve that." Billy Joel's words ring in my head, "Only the good die young!"

As a Christian optimist, I always want to believe people can be healed from all this sickness. I have thought to myself for years, "I wish Jesus were here, on earth, in the flesh again. He would fix these issues. He would heal these little children of all these diseases that are going to keep them from living full lives." The Bible tells us that healing is still a very available part of the

Christian life but that seems so out of reach for most Christians today. It is so difficult to stare into the eyes of medicine and science and historical findings based on facts and figures and say, "I don't accept that! I believe your medical diagnosis may be right, maybe it isn't, what I don't choose to believe is your medical prognosis." Try that a couple of times in the cancer ward at the local hospital and you'll be getting a visit from the onstaff psychiatrist shortly. Fact is, in today's world, you are in the minority if you still believe that God is still in the business of miraculous healing. You are thought of as a "quack" if you walk around quoting Jesus' words about Christians being able to heal the sick, raise the dead and do greater things than He did, and you are among a dying breed. The new way of believing is radically different than that. However, I didn't sit down and put pen to paper to discuss the differences between an older way of believing and a new way of believing. I didn't put pen to paper to convince you of some old, worn out, religious view. I didn't write a word of this to convert you to any particular religion or belief system. In fact, as I will discuss a little later, I didn't even come up with the idea of writing this book. If it is a terrible flop, that's on God, if it is a huge success and even a best seller, that's on God too. I don't have a dog in this fight. Pun intended). The real reason I am writing this is because I was told to. I am also writing this to give you hope. A hope in something different than what you have been told. A hope that somehow, somewhere, there just may be a God who actually cares for you, or your mom or dad, or your spouse or maybe your child. A God who does, in fact, still work miracles. A God who, for whatever reason, occasionally interjects Himself into an equation and renders it scientifically senseless.

I want to share with you about my own experiences and thoughts on this subject. If you vehemently oppose the idea that God could possibly be there, then you may want to stop reading.

However, I hope you do not stop reading, but be forewarned, I cannot tell this story without talking about Him, His actions, what I believe have been His words to me, and what I believe He will do for you. You may not believe a word of this. That has absolutely no effect on its truthfulness. I cannot speak as a scholar, for am not a scholar. Nor can I speak as a saint, or a prophet, for I am neither of these. I can only speak from my heart about what I know is true. I will speak some of what I believe to be true and I will do my best to clarify when I am speaking from factual experience and from speculation and opinion. I ask you not to simply count this as religious mumbo-jumbo and discount the heart touching story I have been given. I ask you to accept the idea that I have been tasked to write to you. And this is to you! The you into whose hands this book has found its way. I have pictured you reading it, have felt your anger, have cried with you the tears of frustration and pain as science has told you what to expect. I have seen you sitting alone in the dark, asking "Why?" I have heard your words as you try to explain the diagnosis to others while your heart breaks again and again to hear the very words come from your own mouth. I don't know you, but I feel you. I want you to know me.

I am Tim and I am going to tell you, mainly, about Winston. Winston and I hope you will stay with us for a while, as we invite you into our lives. It is nice to meet you. We write to you individually. Please, join us as we tell you about ourselves and our story. If you disagree, then let us agree to disagree. Allow us to share with you and hopefully this story will lift your spirit, even if it is just a little. By the way, to all of you English majors out there, I know the "experts" say I shouldn't capitalize all references to God, as in, "He said. His will, He loves us..." but I did, and I am supposed to capitalize satan's name, but, the best way I can put this is... I ain't gonna!

Now, sit back. Put your feet up. Stay a while. Enjoy.

INTRODUCTION

AVAILABLE TOOLS

Let me state firs and foremost; I claim to be nothing special. There is simply nothing exceptional about me, my family, the things we can do for the cause of Christ, or our particular relationship with God The Father. We are normal people. We do not claim to have special gifts or a special anything. We have our faults, fears, temptations, and weaknesses. We do not practice any particular level of holiness other than that which we feel called to be and even in those callings, we fail often. We are human and nothing greater than humans with the exception that we have answered the call to live for Christ and therefore, we are children of God with Christ living in us. Even with that said, very often I feel I am the least of humans upon which God should call. I find it baffling at times, that He would even consider using me.

I am a woodworker by nature, and the only sense I can make of God actually using me is in this comparison;

occasionally, in my woodworking, I go to the tool box and dig out a rusty old tool that hasn't been used for years, go to the grinding wheel or sanding belt, sharpen said tool to the best of my ability, (usually I have to oil it considerably, because of rust) then I put it to use, for it is, at the moment, the tool I have at my disposal, for the job. It is not likely the best tool for the job. It is likely not the only tool I have that could perform the task at hand. It is simply the tool I have which I have chosen, at the specific moment, for the specific job. It is available. It is able to be sharpened. It may appear old and worn out and it may have been designed for a completely different job all together. However, at the moment, for the specific work I have, it works and I will use it. This is the only feasible reason I can find that God would even consider calling me to a specific task. I am available, I will do what He asks, most of the time. I work therefore, He will use me.

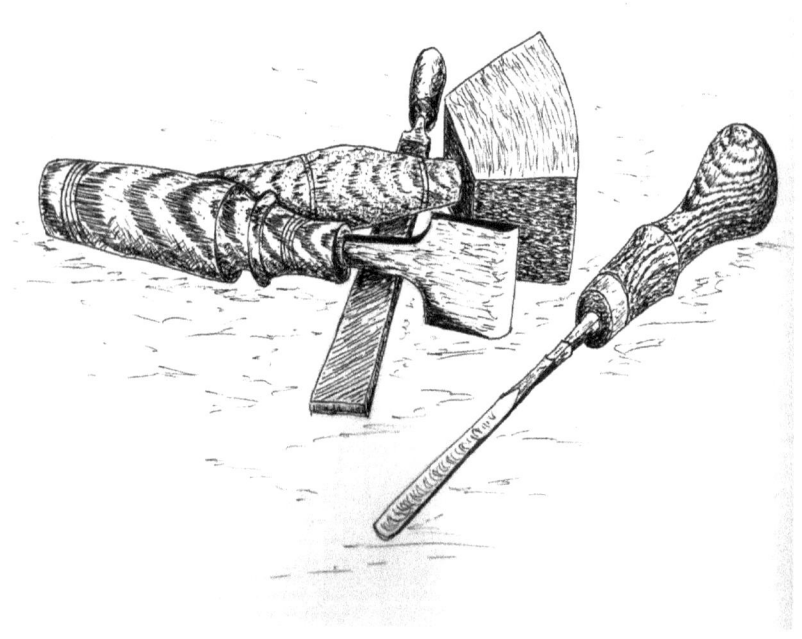

Allow me to make a side note here while we are getting to know each other. Among other things, I am also a hunter. I have no idea how some of my readers may feel about the subject of hunting. I understand we may have vastly different opinions about this. Please do not dismiss this work because we believe differently. There are parts of this story that may reference this aspect of my life because Winston is, in fact, a hunting dog as well as a family pet. We can agree to disagree on whether hunting is necessary or even ethical, but to entirely dismiss this work would be a great dis-service to us all. The Winston Story is not about hunting at all. The Story is about a dog, his sickness, our trials together, how it relates to my life and hopefully how it may relate to yours. We have this one thing in common, no matter where we are on any level of political correctness; We are all doing life and at times, life can really stink. "The Story" is about just that. Life. Having said that, allow me to further explain. This Story begins with a lot of disassociated parts and it rambles around. The reader may come to the conclusion because of all of the incongruity, the partial stories laid out before you,"This writer is a buffoon!" Stay with me. God is an amazing weaver of stranded web. In light of that, I begin where it all began.

Habakkuk 2:2-3

2. Then the Lord answered me and said:

"Write the vision
And make it plain on tablets,
That he may run who reads it.

3.   For the vision is yet for an appointed time;

But at the end it will speak, and it will not lie.

Though it tarries, wait for it;
Because it will surely come,
It will not tarry.

ONE

DOGS

I have owned Labrador Retrievers since I was about 20 years old, often owning several at a time. I have always had at least one. I have trained them on a semi-professional level since my late 20's and have owned the same bloodline for about 28 years. I received my first yellow lab as a gift from a working associate and named him Drake. Over the years, Drake sired many litters and one of his female puppies went to a duck hunting friend of mine. When Drake died at 14 years old, that friend of mine had a litter of puppies from the female he had received from me. He called me with interesting news and told me there was one puppy in the entire litter which was colored exactly like Drake. As far as my friend was concerned, that puppy belonged to me. We called him "Woody" which is short for "Wood duck" in hunter's terms, and he filled an empty void in my life that was left by losing his grandfather, Drake. He continued to fill voids as my life took an ugly turn that resulted in divorce. Woody, for a long time, was all I had that resembled family. Ultimately, my daughter, Ashley, came to live with me, but for a while, it was just me and ole' Woody, doing life together.

I began a new chapter in my life when I met Karen. She was the most incredible person I may have ever known, and an amazing creature. Wise beyond her years, with a soft heart for the needy and a pliable mind for God's purposes. She is not perfect, in the same regard that none of mankind is perfect, yet she is a much better person than I. I truly understand how He could see promise and unlimited potential in her. She may disagree, but I see her with a different eye than almost anyone else, and with that, I can imagine how He must see her, knowing her depths better than she knows herself. It was, in all those lovely characteristics that I see, that I fell deeply in love with her. She has two daughters, Kaitlyn and Abby, and of course, Ashley was living with me and there was Jonathan, my son, who was attending college. She is 11 years younger than I am so her girls, of course, are quite a bit younger than my kids. We both had baggage and issues. We loved each other wonderfully and the girls got along great. We all loved being together, every moment we could, so marriage seemed to be the best answer for that. So, in May of 2009, somehow, I convinced her to marry me and we joined our families together under one roof.

Woody, as I stated, was a huge part of my life. He was 88 lbs. of excited yellow lab that was geared for duck and goose hunting. When Karen entered my life, he and my daughter came with me as a package deal and she embraced the three of us into her life, dog hair and all. After about a year of marriage we began to discuss getting another dog and my thoughts were to get a female Lab. We were thinking of finding a silver lab for breeding purposes but when we began looking, Karen stumbled across a "discount puppy" we simply could not resist. She found a German Short-haired Pointer pup, who was the last one left in the litter. I had always wanted a "GSP" and she had been marked down considerably from her original price and was only about 20 miles away. We decided to go take a look. That night, "Heidi" became part of our family and a friendship was made with her owner, Chris McDaniel.

Heidi had one of the best personalities I had ever experienced. She immediately began her work at the house as a pointer and was doing very well. It was early in the year and we had lots of time to train before hunting season. We had some very unfavorable weather that March and so I didn't train much until mid April. When we resumed our training, Heidi was suddenly gun shy. I assume that the crazy lightning storms we had been having had turned her inside out and there was no convincing her that the sound would not hurt her. My dreams were crushed a bit but she had firmly rooted her character into our family and there was no turning back on that either! So, we had a neurotic, gun shy, GSP who only pointed lizards and frogs who loved our family with an immeasurable passion. A couple years later we found out we couldn't breed her to raise puppies because she had a rare condition. So, we had a neurotic, gun shy, GSP who only pointed lizards and frogs and could not be bred... who loved our family with an immeasurable passion. Over a short period of time, we also realized she was horrified of storms. To the point that she tried to eat her way out of a room through the wall and door, once, while we were not home. So,we had a neurotic, gun shy, GSP who only pointed lizards and frogs and could not be bred and was horrified of lightning...who loved our family with an immeasurable passion. Next, she grew terribly resistant to being locked up in any fashion. She destroyed all manner of things. She destroyed chain-linked fencing, metal wire kennels, literally anything that contained her. She ate her way through the side of a plastic kennel! She simply would not be locked anywhere, for any time, without losing it. So, we had a neurotic, gun shy, GSP who only pointed lizards and frogs and could not be bred and was horrified of lightning and could not be locked into a cage.... who loved our family with an immeasurable passion. She was such a blessing. There was a fleeting moment in her life when I took her, in spite of my better judgment, to a pheasant shoot to collect downed birds. I was astonished to see that all the bird action had her ignoring the gun shots completely. She was quite old for a new training, by this time, but she took to it fairly well. In the lunch break, she and I headed off to the tall grass to see if we could find one of the few pheasant that had escaped the guns of the crowd. Moments in, she "locked up" on point and although she crept forward and flushed it, she had given me enough time to close the gap well enough to kill the bird on the jump. She didn't bolt at the shot and she ran to see it downed. When she reached the bird she seemed to recoil a bit at the scent of it and refused to pick it up. Rather, she bolted off to find yet another live bird. I never got close enough to the second one before she had it up and flying off into yonder woods, but she had fulfilled a life time dream for me and was proud of doing so. She came back and pranced around for having scared off such a terrible creature and that was it. That was the extent of my upland bird hunting over Heidi.

WINSTON THE WONDER DOG

In an attempt for expediency, I will not go into the boring details of how he became part of our family. I will just say, due to a long standing dog-trading agreement I mentioned before, with the same old friend, we acquired the third male yellow lab of my life. I wanted to name him "Decoy" but my dear wife in all of her wisdom, told me that was not his name. "Winchester" was his name. So, he became "Woody's little Winchester" officially, "Winston" for short. Let me make something clear, that is Winston as in Winston Churchill, not the cigarette. Winston, the grandson of Woody, who was the grandson of Drake, came to live with us in the spring of 2014. He showed promise of being the best retriever I had ever owned, as Woody began to live out his retirement from waterfowl retrieving. Two years later Woody, at 13 yrs old, went to the great "waterfowling hole in the sky," and Winston and Heidi were all we had left.

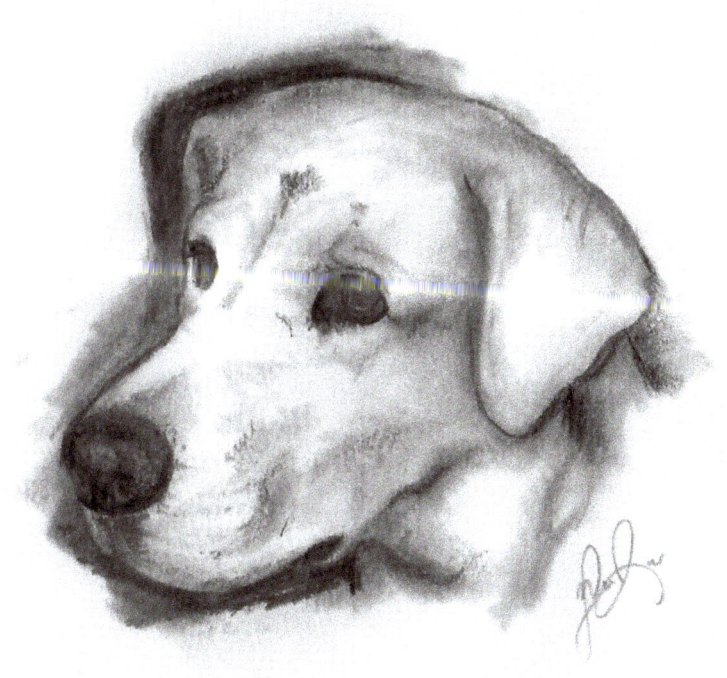

WOODIE'S LITTLE WINCHESTER
AKA
"WINSTON"

TWO

RAIS~A~RUCKUS

I mentioned the new friendship I gained with Chris, the litter owner from which we obtained Heidi. Chris and I hit it off well and because of that, we started hunting together occasionally. On one hunting trip Chris had a catastrophic moment and ended up turning over his canoe in deep water. It was about 28 degrees that morning and while Chris clung to the bottom of his canoe in the frigid waters, I did all I could do to sprint, in my waders, through a swamp, to get to another boat. When I finally reached Chris he had kicked to the opposite shore but was laying on his back, half in-half out of the water at the edge of the lake. He was alive but he was quite gray in color, shivering terribly and clearly in the onset stages of hypothermia. I righted the canoe and somehow, got Chris into the bottom of it . I wrapped him in my dry coat and had him hold his dog against his chest (dogs' body temps are greater than ours) and paddled him to his mother's house.

Chris survived just fine, but was so grateful that he insisted I take his duck call that he had made for himself. It is a beautiful piece of artwork made from spalted Hickory and I loved it, although I still think he was silly for insisting upon my taking it. As silly as it may have seemed to me at the time, I had no idea that it would spark in me the desire to start making my own duck calls, but it did. And from that, started Rais~A~Ruckus Game Calls. I started making custom made duck and goose calls and selling them through stores and over the internet. The company grew quickly and people started recognizing me as the "duck call guy" around town.

Owning a duck call company, especially during the height of the "Duck Dynasty phenomenon" was kind of cool. Our first event was a wild game dinner at Bethlehem First Baptist church in Bethlehem, Ga. One of the only calls we sold that night was to a young man named Anderson and his step father named John. Anderson proved to be a huge asset as he began to sell my calls at his high-school and he became my first "prostaff" member. John, his step father, quickly turned into a friend of mine and was clearly a strong Christian. John is one of those guys who knows so much scripture you can say almost anything to him about almost any subject and he will know a scripture that applies to it. Often, we would end a conversation and I would walk away shaking my head thinking, "That dude is WILD."

The second event we attended was a large trade show and on the first night, right before closing, a pastor came by our booth. We talked for a while and to my surprise he had asked me to come to his church and speak to his men's group and tell my story/testimony. I did. It was a great experience that sparked in me a desire to share my story and before long I had several invitations for speaking engagements.

LISTENING TO THE VOICE OF GOD

One very cold morning, strangely enough, during a training session with Winston, God showed me a new comparison that I could share with others. As I was training Winston, I noticed he was paying very close attention to me. His intensity about watching my every move was amazing. He could read my body language almost like he could read my mind. He had paid such close attention to me that he knew what I would ask of him based on the training scenario. In the midst of training, I believe I heard God speak to me. "Why don't you pay attention to me with that kind of intesity?" "Whoa!" I thought, "Where did that come from? I thought I DID pay attention to you!" I stood there on the side of the pond, with great conviction overcoming me, and I apologized for not listening with intensity. I told Him I wanted to hear and know His voice better. I made a new commitment to lean in and listen. Then, I went back to training.

There was ice on the side of the pond, and Winston had to break it with each retrieve. I knew that water had to be incredibly cold on his young body, but Winston didn't care. He was doing what he loved and would come out of the water with joy to deliver the retrieving bumper so he could do it again. As the steam boiled from his wet fur in the fridged air, his eyes beamed with excitment. I marvelled at my one-year-old Lab's enthusiasm. Rarely, had I seen a pup with that level of drive! Then, quietly, deep within my heart, I heard The Lord speak again. "And, when I ask you to do things, why don't you do them with that much joy, regardless of the circumstances?"

Ouch. That stung a little, maybe a lot. I could get on board with listening intently to His voice, that would benefit me as much as anyone else. Being able to "hear God's voice" would be a great thing for anyone. But this, this hurt. I sat down on the side of the pond in my waders. The soaked dog ran over to me with the bumper in his mouth. I am sure he wondered why dad was crying. I am sure he just wanted to play fetch a little more. He sat down holding the bumper proudly hoping that would get me back into the game. I was wrecked. I knew that I had engaged in complaining or grumbling about some aspects of ministry. It's not always a bowl of cherries. People take advantage of you at times. Other times, you simply go unappreciated. Often, the hours are long, the pay, if any, is little, and the outcomes are depressing. It is always a heavy thing to be reminded that Christ went to the cross for us, with far more pain and abandonment than we will ever know. As I rubbed the wet head of my pup, through the tears, I asked for His forgiveness again and recommitted to working for Him with new-found joy.

That was enough training for me that day! I couldn't take more lessons if that was the way they were going to go. I loaded up the truck and headed home. On the way home, I believe He sat with me in the truck and opened my eyes to another thing. I could take Winston, do a retrieving demonstration and share with others this new message of "Listening intently to the voice of God and doing what He asked with joy, regardless of the circumstances." How could I resist? It was a great opportunity to make others feel as bad as He had made me feel!! And with that new message Winston was launched, merely a year old, into ministry. He would go with me and be a demonstration and an example for men and youth. We were often invited to speak in churches in our area.

The next year we began, with Rais~A~Ruckus, attending a festival in the small town, Hoschton, GA. Their fall festival is a three day event that also hosts a dock diving competition for dogs. If you have never seen one of these, it is quite a spectacle. Basically, they install a temporary pool of sorts, with a dock attached to one end. The pool has measured hash-marks down the sides for ease of measuring the length of jumps by the dogs. The "handler" which is a fancy name for the person who is directing the dog, holds the dog back and tosses a retrieving bumper into the long narrow pool. By various means of getting the dog excited, the handler then releases the dog from the back of the dock. The dog runs down the dock and leaps into the water to fetch said bumper and where the base of the tail of the dog enters the water, the dog's measured "leap" is recorded and the competition goes from there. The dogs that usually do the best are large, strong, agile and athletic dogs that typically have a lean body style. Think greyhound style animals. However, they also need a natural desire to be strong fetching animals to increase the drive. Some of the best in the world are Belgian Malinois. These have, in recent years, become the go-to animals for drug dogs and protection dogs. They are hard driving, super fast, athletic animals, yet very lean with the natural fetching instinct that matches any Labrador Retriever I have ever seen. Their greatest advantage over a lab, in the dock diving world, is the fact they weigh about a third less than a lab of the same stature. They are naturally strong and very driven. They usually have long legs and therefore, they are naturally going to be able to jump further than another dog with the same muscle mass, such as a Lab. Our daughter, Abby, fell in love with the idea of taking Winston to the Dock Diving competition and entering him. He had a lot of drive, that's for sure, and he loved to leap into the water after his retrieving bumpers, so, we decided to give it a shot.

A few days before the competition, I decided to take him to a friend's house who had a pond with a dock and train a little. He did very well from what I could tell but I had no way to measure his jumps and no idea of how the other dogs would perform.

The morning of the competition, Abby took Winston over

to the pool for a few trial jumps and to get her bearings on how she could excite him the most before releasing him to make his jumps. His practice jumps landed him in the water at about 15 feet. The people running the event said that was pretty good for a first timer and we discussed how to get him more riled up and some other techniques for tossing the bumper.

When competition time rolled around we were nervous, but excited for her and Winston. On his first jump the new technique seemed to be a good decision. On his second jump he earned a new name. "Winston the Wonder Dog" flew 22 feet, 4 inches. It took him into a new category, which in reality, wasn't a great thing for scoring against his competition. The thing that was incredible about this jump was that he was carrying 98 lbs of Labrador Retriever through the air for that distance! His strongest competition was a Malinois who had been doing this for years who only weighed about 65 lbs. Abby and Winston won second place overall in the competition and first place in the youth handler's bracket. Our yellow boy could fly! They competed for two years at the festival and he scored pretty much the same both years.

THREE

CONNECTIONS

RESTORATION CHURCH

In the same year that Winston came to live with us, Karen went to work with a new Orthodontist. Her new work family seemed to be a bunch of great gals. She started with the new doctor a few weeks before Christmas. The annual Christmas party was scheduled and husbands were invited. We showed up, not knowing what to expect and ended up sitting next to a couple of youngsters that seemed quite nice. James and Jessica talked with us through the evening and we found quite a bit of common ground. It seemed obvious they were Christians and soon the talk turned to where everyone was going to church. We were sort of "in the market" as they say, for a new place to worship and they invited us to come hear a preacher who was being considered as a pastor for their church. Travis Rutland was his name. I happened to know of Travis as I had followed his father, Dr. Mark Rutland, for years. I told Karen I was very interested in hearing Travis speak and it was decided that we would go. We have not been to another church since. Over the last 5 years, my Christian walk has matured so much under Travis and we are now serving on staff at the church. In the spring of 2017, Travis asked Karen and I to accept an interim position as youth directors. I had been praying about doing ministry work again, and had hoped that I could work with the men of the church or maybe in missions or something like that. I had never, not once, considered or hoped for a position of working with teens. So when Travis asked if we would do that, we were both somewhat reluctant. However, God was calling and we felt compelled to answer. So youth minister it was. We hit the ground running with the youth department and the pieces began to come together and before we knew it, we were thoroughly enjoying what we were doing. Around the end of the year, Travis hired a young man and his wife, Tyler and Megan Ellis. They started their time with Restoration Church as Children's Ministers. Tyler beamed with energy and dreams and fit well into our staff. At the beginning of February, 2018 Tyler came to me with a question.

HAITI

"Don't you have a construction background?" Tyler asked. After informing him of all I used to do, he said I would be perfect to fill a need. He was apparently part of a mission organization that was building an orphanage in Haiti. He needed someone to go and take a look at some construction that had been partially completed thus far, and advise them on the quality of what had been done and what to do next. He and Megan were going and wanted Karen and I to go with them. The Missions organization would pick up the tab and it would only be a short trip, out and back in 3 days.

We decided to accompany them and off we went to Haiti.

14

We were *not prepared* for Haiti.

It is a little overwhelming. It was busy. It was a little scary. It was dirty and poor. It was unlike any third world country I had ever visited... Yet, the children, ohh the children, they were both heart warming and heartbreaking at the same time. The need in Haiti is vast. Imagine someone taking on the task of filling a great crater, hundreds of feet wide and deep with dirt, ordering dump trucks full of dirt and standing at the side of the crater, throwing dirt over the crater's edge, one shovelful at a time. That is what it feels like to think of taking on a task in Haiti to me. However, one shovelful equals one child's heart at a time, so each shovelful counts.

Karen's heart was torn for the children there. She wanted to bring them home by the dozens. I think she began to be able to see herself doing some kind of mission work at that moment. Maybe not in Haiti, but somewhere, doing God's work. It was exciting to see the work God was doing in her.

TLCB and D

In February 2018, we were also presented with an opportunity to take over a franchise of a small advertising business. It is called; The Little Coupon Book (TLCB). It is exactly that, a little book of various advertisements for local stores, from restaurants to local contractors and full, end to end, of different types of coupons. One of the main preceptsof selling ads for TLCB is to build relationships with your customers. Throughout the year I had begun to do just that. One of which was a small boutique in Monroe, GA that had been running an ad in our book for a few months. The manager, my main contact, was a young lady, in her late 30's. We will refer to her as "D". She was nice and friendly, and we had worked together while attempting to attract more people to her store.

The last month they were running an ad with us, I was under a lot of pressure to sell some new ads. I had planned to go to Winder, a neighboring city, but it seemed as though everything I was trying to accomplish before I headed that way, was simply not going to happen in time. It was as if I was walking through wet concrete. Everything took twice as long as it should that day and I was never going to make Winder. So, with a couple more hours of work available to me, I decided to stay in Monroe and call on some of my present customers. I parked at the north end of Broad street and headed south down the sidewalk. I popped in on D first. Regardless of the fact, she had told me days before they were probably going to try some other type of advertising the next month, I was compelled to drop by for some reason. The shop was empty with the exception of her, standing behind the checkout counter as I made my way to the back of the store.

"How are you young lady?" I asked.

"Well, I've been better."

I noticed she was upset, it seemed to be all over her. I didn't want to pry into her business but for some reason my heart went out to her.

"What's going on D?" I inquired.

"I went to the Eye Doctor this morning. He told me I have a disease that will render me blind within ten years," she said flatly. "Tim, I'm young. So by the time I'm like 48 I may be completely blind. On top of that, basically, they say there's no cure."

I don't really know what came over me. Something between compassionate hope and anger, strangely welled up in me. I stood there for a moment trying to take it in. Something in me wanted to argue. Something else in me thought, "You're crazy, and if you say what you're thinking, she is going to know you're crazy." Yet, I couldn't help myself.

"No you're not going to be blind, D," I started, "I can't

explain why I feel this way, but I just don't believe that is what God has in store for you."

There…it was out. My mind was reeling because I had just declared something that could give her a lot of false hope and make me look quite crazy. "This is serious stuff, Tim," I thought, and although I felt strongly that she would not be blind, I had to remind myself, "You're talking to a woman about her eyesight… this isn't a common cold!"

"I believe," I continued, "that God had me come here today for a reason! I'm not even supposed to be here, I am supposed to be in Winder! Think about the timing and all the things that had to fall into place to make this happen at this very moment. God loves you that much and He made it 'just-so-happen' for me to be in your store at this moment so we could talk privately and you could share your pain with me. I want to pray with you. Can we do that?"

She agreed and we prayed. I told her I would come back so we could talk more. When I left, honestly, I felt half crazy and a little scared. But, I still believe God is healing D's eyesight.

17

FOUR

CEREBRAL DISEQUILIBRIUM

I f you have ever hydroplaned in a car, especially while behind the wheel, you will be able to relate to this feeling. As you are driving, you suddenly become distinctly aware of the disconnect between your tires and the pavement. This is usually onset by driving too fast for the present conditions. However, "why" you are spinning becomes less and less important as time slows down and seconds are split into micro-seconds. You can remember having distinct thoughts, that later on, take much longer to relay than it took to think them, as you began to spin. You hold on to the steering wheel and your mind goes into over-drive trying to compensate for the chaos evolving around you. In most cases, you are truly helpless. You can only hang on and hope this ends well. Occasionally, life spins us like this. We realize we are completely out of control of anything and we are simply along for the ride. Our emotional sense of balance disintegrates and we are there to observe the chaos, with no ability to reign it in. I call that "cerebral disequilibrium."

MEANWHILE, AT MY HOME

As you are aware, we are a dog family. We love having them around (most times) and love the companionship. Winston and Heidi lived indoors with us and have been as much of the family as we are ourselves. Heidi with all of her issues, was one of the sweetest pets I have ever been around. She loved everything about being with us and once we got used to living around her neurotic behavior, she was never again a problem. Winston was proving to be the hardest driving, most energetic working dog I had ever owned. After Abby began working with him in the dock dog competitions he also finished his first retriever test with ease. He wasn't just a working dog though, he was proving to be an incredible family pet as well. We could not move about the house without Winston matching our steps, simply wanting to be near us. He and Heidi played with their toys together and were bonded so tightly it was heart warming to watch them. Never have I seen two dogs more close to one another and to the members of their family. As the grey grew more prevalent across Heidi's muzzle we feared for Winston's level of heart ache when the inevitable came to be. In June of 2018, our worries increased.

Almost simultaneously, Heidi began to show signs of some kind of bladder issue and Winston began to limp on his right foot a little. Having raised and trained dogs for nearly 30 years, I have seen a myriad of health issues. Therefore, we decided first, to take the home remedy approach. We began treating Heidi with Cranberry Juice, which she drank for a few days. She then became quite picky about what she was going to drink. I began by suspending Winston's retrieving, believing the cause for his limping was a strained front, right shoulder. I had checked all the obvious possibilities, cut feet, briers, etc. The pain seemed to be more in the shoulder and as hard as he always worked, I felt confident he just needed to rest for a while.

Over a period of a couple weeks, Heidi's condition seemed to worsen slightly and Winston would get better for a day or two and then begin to limp again. We would watch Heidi squat to urinate and she couldn't finish. She would stop. Take a few steps, and then squat again. Finally, we decided to call the mobile vet out to the house. Dr. A. showed up the next day to take a urine sample and examine her. She felt it was likely nothing major and while she was at the house she took a look at Winston's shoulder. She agreed with my original diagnosis and prescribed an anti-inflammatory medicine, as well as a mild sedative to help him rest in the indoor kennel. A few days later the test results came back, we discussed Heidi's issues. The bladder was not infected as we thought, rather, she was suffering from one of two problems. Either a psychoneurosis issue thinking she was thirsty all the time and forcing her to need to urinate quite often or a major problem with her kidneys. We treated her for the psychosis first, trying to eliminate that possibility.

Meanwhile, Winston continued his "on again, off again" condition. Heidi seemed to get a little better while we limited her water intake but then worsened once more. Frustration began to build as we were doing pretty much all we could afford to do and neither of them seemed to be getting much better. We talked once again to the Dr and in early August she prescribed total kennel rest for Winston. He was completely restricted to his kennel while Heidi seemed to be doing the same or worse week by week.

THE VET

Around the 24th of August I called Dr A. once again, and described Winston's condition as the same. We all agreed we needed to have an X-ray done of his shoulder. I had been speaking about the problem with my sister and she recommended we use a particular vet who was supposed to be trained in the art of acupuncture for animals. Thinking the problem was muscular or ligament or tendon related, I thought this may be a good idea. I made an appointment with her for Tuesday, August 28th. They took us to the room and he limped around and hopped back to the X-ray room with the assistant. They left me there for a short while as I worked through some business issues on my phone. The assistant returned, looking a little concerned, and asked if I would follow her to the back because the Dr. wanted to show me the x-rays. As I entered the room I could see what was obviously Winston's front legs and chest on the digital screen in front of the doctor. She was sitting in a chair looking at the screen.

"Well, what's up?" I asked.

She looked over her shoulder at me and I could see on her face, she was seriously concerned about her findings. "It's bad." she said, flatly.

Startled at her lack of bedside manner, I stopped and stared. "What does that mean?" I asked.

"He has bone cancer." She said flatly.

Honestly, my memory cannot truly recall what else she said at that moment. I can remember moving closer to the screen and being shown the large lesion on his upper right humerus. I asked if I could photograph it. I planned to send it immediately to my long-time friend/vet, Keith Cox in North Ga. Frankly, I thought, "This lady is a quack! There's no way he has cancer! He's only 4 years old, how could he have cancer?" She continued to talk to me but it was as if she was talking to me from down a hall, just far enough away that I could hear her voice but could not distinguish the words. She sent me back to the room and said she would be there in a few minutes.

I tried to call Karen and she didn't pick up. I made the terrible mistake of simply shooting her the findings in a text. "they say he has bone cancer." What an idiot I was, sending that kind of news through a text! Immediately, I received a phone call and I answered to the sound of her crying on the other end. We were both in disbelief. I sent the text to Keith and it only took a few minutes for him to respond in sorrow. His words were, "I am sorry friend. I have to agree with her diagnosis. You are up against a very hard spot." They emailed the x-rays to Keith for me and they also reached out to the Oncology Department of the school of veterinarian education, at a local, south-eastern university. The head of the department spoke with our vet and they all agreed; bone cancer, very aggressive, and very advanced.

Karen and I were speaking on the phone and as the vet was coming into the room, I told Karen, "I feel like I should pray. But, I don't even know if you can pray for your dog...I don't even know if it is appropriate to believe that God will heal your dog....does God even *do dogs*?" I asked. Before you get too judgy on me, I couldn't recall anytime in the Bible where someone's animal was healed. I know we *can pray* about anything. But I just didn't know, for sure, if it was appropriate to believe in the miraculous healing power of God for your dog.

Then I continued with Karen, "Let me see what she has to say and I will call you back." As we were ending the call, God spoke into my mind like an arrow shot from heaven.

FIVE

THE PROMISE

A complete memory in an instant. A confirmation of what God "does and doesn't do." I had not thought of Randy in years. His story went something like, "Somehow, my guitar, which was a gift from my wife, got scratched. It was scratched badly. As in, you could run your fingernail along it and feel the recess." The guitar was a solid black, very expensive guiar and apparently, you could see the scratch very well. Randy was clearly upset about the scratch and decided to pray about it. Suddenly, for whatever reason, he felt like God spoke to him about the scratch. "Go and pray over your guitar and rub the scratch," God said to him, according to Randy. He relayed the story on a Sunday morning with tears in his eyes and a crack in his voice. He repeated it to me a few weeks ago as I inquired of him to ensure my memory was correct. He went into his study and picked up the guitar, prayed, and began to rub the scratch with a cloth. "Now, this wasn't like a mark or a transfer of paint, it was scratched deeply." He recounted to me. "But to my amazement," he continued, "the scratch simply began to go away. In a few minutes, you could no longer feel it and a few more minutes the surface of the guitar appeared as if nothing had ever happened." It may have been 15 years since I had even thought of Randy's guitar, yet, there it was in my mind in full detail. In what seemed like a fraction of a second, the entire story replayed while I stood there in the Vet's office as she began to speak to me.

"I spoke again with the oncology department at the university….."

I tried to listen to her as I began to hear God's voice, "**If I cared enough about a man and his guitar...**"

"They said you could bring him there and they could start radiation and chemotherapy treatment immediately. The cost would be somewhere between 10 and 12,000 dollars," the vet was explaining.

"**Then I care enough about a man and his dog.**" His voice drowned out the sound of her talking.

"However, they felt that would only give Winston about a year to live. I spoke to them about aggressive removal of the leg, all the way up to the ball joint, and they felt like that would only give you a few months." the Vet somberly explained.

I could hear what she was saying but I was trying to process what I felt God had just said. "**If I cared enough about a man and his guitar...Then I care enough about a man and his dog.**"

"What was that supposed to mean," I wondered. "God, does that mean you're going to heal Winston or that you just care about the fact he is dying?"

I felt my eyes begin to fill with tears. I didn't want to show that kind of emotion. I could see Winston in my mind. I could see Abby sending him down the ramp at the dock diving competition. I could see him barreling through the tall grass fetching at the pheasant shoots. I could see the dirt flying up from behind him as he tore away from me when I gave him his favorite command, "Fetch!" I could see him running, as the girls in my family encouraged the raucous behavior, "Go Wincy Go!" they would shout as he ran with his butt tucked low under him, as fast as he could, from the closet, through the bathroom, to a flying leap onto our bed. Doing what I called "the low-butt run". I could see him bounding through 10 inches of water, fetching a dead duck that was just shot over a rice field. I could see him diving into nearly frozen ponds to swim 80 yards to pick up a Canada Goose. I could not picture any of those things with him missing a front leg all the way to the shoulder. All I could see, when she said that, was a poor, discouraged, depressed Winston, laying on the floor watching me get ready to go hunting. He would hop along after me as I walked through the house preparing all of my gear. I could see his begging eyes stare at me as I closed the door between us. I would walk to the truck and he would hop across the room to lay on the floor beside Karen's chair.

The statement just lay there, in my mind, like a fact. "**If I cared enough about a man and his guitar…Then I care enough about a man and his dog.**"

"I'm not doing that to Winston." I replied. "I just don't know what to do or think. What would you do?" I asked her flatly. My mind was still trying to get wrapped around what she was saying and what I thought I heard God saying.

"Well, if he were mine, there would be no question, I would be on my way to start Chemotherapy. But not everyone can do that." She answered.

"Yeah, that's not really an option for me." I quipped, realizing that we were obviously speaking from two different financial platforms, as well as two different platforms of reality.

"Unfortunately," she continued, "even if you do choose

to do one of these, this cancer is very advanced and very aggressive,"

....."**If I cared enough about a man and his guitar...Then I care enough about a man and his dog.**"

"... you're only going to extend his life for a relatively short period of time. But, aside from these two treatment plans, I'm sorry Mr. Rupard, you don't really have any good options..."

The two statements echoe in my head to this day. "...You don't really have any good options.." "**If I cared enough about a man and his guitar...Then I care enough about a man and his dog.**" "I'm sorry Mr. Rupard, aside from these two treatment plans...you don't have any other options...." "**If I cared enough about a man and his guitar...**"

There was a battle going on for my mind.

"...don't have any other options.." "......**Then I care enough about a man and his dog.**"

"...no other options..." "**If I cared enough..Then I care enough...**"

"He cares enough..." rang through my spirit. "He cares enough." it got louder and louder in my head, welling up from somewhere deep within me. "HE CARES ENOUGH!!!!!"

The vet continued, "I'm going to have our office manager come in and talk to you about some financial issues while you think about it."

I cut her off mid-sentence, "Well, I am not going to take his leg off, Winston is simply too full of life for me to do that to him. I cannot afford to do the university thing....I think I have another option." I said.

That statement stopped her in her tracks as she had turned to leave the room. She turned around and looked at me inquisitively.

I continued, "Frankly, this may seem crazy to you but I don't think he's going to die. I believe God is going to heal

Winston."

There. I had said it. My mind was reeling with confusion. First, I was wondering how my 4 year old lab had bone cancer. Especially bone cancer that was advanced. Second, I was wondering how my family was going to get through this. This dog meant everything to us. He had been such a huge part of our lives, how was this going to happen? Third, I was wondering how I could be standing there with any faith at all, let alone enough to deny a scientific fact; He had terminal bone cancer. I wondered just how preposterous it was for me to be saying, "No! That doesn't work for us!" Fourth, where was this coming from? Was it me just being hard headed or was this actually coming from God? I believed I heard God say, "If I care enough about a man and his guitar, then I care enough about a man and his dog." Word for word, that's what I felt like I heard. But that didn't mean I heard Him say, "I'm going to heal Winston." It just meant I heard that He *cared enough* to heal him.

The vet looked at me as if I were a pitifully confused soul and said something like (and I say "something like" because in my mental turmoil, I wasn't exactly listening to every word she said), "Well, in times like these, very often, people turn to their faith to help themselves. There is nothing wrong with that, if that is what makes you feel better. My office manager will be in to talk to you about your bill." With that, she turned and left the room. My sister, Angela, had told me she didn't know if the vet was a believer or not. Angela had said the vet had made a few comments, over the years, which led my sister to believe that she may not have been. My mind was shocked to hear her say those words so bluntly to me but I quickly caught myself and knew that it wasn't the time for a theological debate. It didn't matter what either of us said at the moment anyway. I simply believed that God was going to heal him and no one was going to sway that belief. I couldn't explain my stubborn belief, I still cannot explain it. It just came to me there in the examination room, and it hasn't left me since.

I left that office with belief in my heart and doubts in my head. The battle that was raging between the two was intense. All my analytical senses were telling me I was a fool for even considering that science wasn't perfectly correct. In fact, science *was* correct in one sense. The bone cancer was as obvious as the sun or a mountain range. All you had to do was to look at the photograph. Like a photo of a sunset or a mountain range, seeing is believing. The mountains are as real as real can be. Even if you lived in a sleepy little coastal town and had never left your home to see anything other than flat coastal land, the reality of a mountain range doesn't change. I have never laid eyes on Mount Everest, but I have seen the photos and I am 100 percent convinced it is real. Those photos are proof. My mind saw the lesion on the x-rays that the Vet pointed to when she said "That's bone cancer, and it's advanced." My mind clearly understood Keith's message when I read, "Unfortunately, I agree with her assessment, you guys are in a tough spot, my friend, I am sorry." Clearly, I believe the Vet actually talked with the head of the Oncology Department at the local university as she claimed she did. He verified her suspicions with his own diagnosis of bone cancer and added that it was "aggressive and advanced." There was simply no doubt about the opinions of science, when it came to what we were all seeing. However, there was something else burning inside of me, something that refused to budge, something that pushed back at all the sensible ideas. Was this what it felt like for the blind man, when Jesus spit on the ground, made a paste of dirt and saliva, rubbed it onto his closed eyes and told him to go to the pool of Siloam and wash it all off? When he walked away, the mud covering his eyes beginning to dry and crack, wandering towards the pool, he must have been thinking, "God, I hope this works!" It had to be running through his mind, "What if this guy is just a crack job? What are all the people going to say about me? They are already mean enough to me! Oh, how they must be prepared to laugh their heads off...I'm going to look ten times the fool they already say I am... I mean, I've heard crazy things about this Jesus before, stories of healing, stories of miracles, but I have never stood in the face of science to defy all logic! God, I hope I was right in standing up and asking for healing! God, I hope he is right for sending me on my way like this... God, I hope the waters in the pool work!"

As I left the Vet's office, I felt foolish. I remember lifting Winston into the back seat of the truck. They had told me the leg was fragile. The bone walls were already very thin. They explained, that the walls would continue to thin and eventually the leg would break. At that point, the cancer would be released into his bloodstream and spread very quickly, not to mention, he would be in incredible pain. It would be at this moment we would need to be prepared to make the decision to put him down. My imagination was running wild. I wanted it all to be a bad dream. I spoke to Karen again and filled her in on the details the vet shared with me. After speaking to her for a bit, she had to go back to work. I called my sister, Angela again. I wanted her to know what the vet had told me, but more than anything I just wanted to talk to someone. I told her of what I believed God had said. Angela was filled with faith and supported me, but she gave me some strict admonition.

"If you're going to ask something like this (Winston's healing) from God, You're gonna have to show Him you are serious," she warned me.

" What do you mean?" I inquired.

"I think you need to fast and pray, if you are going to ask God to heal him." Angela directed.

I had never fasted before, but, it was as if Jesus had

31

simply sat down in the truck and said, "I want you to fast." In retrospect, I may have been grasping at anything that I could do to try and push God into doing what I wanted Him to do. Even so, I felt strongly that Angela was right. If I was going to get serious with God about what I wanted Him to do, I needed to show Him I was serious about it as well. I had felt as if God had spoken to me, I needed to be focused for whatever it was He was about to do. I had eaten breakfast that morning but I knew immediately I wouldn't have lunch or dinner. I decided instantaneously, "Yes, I will fast."

The rest of the day is a blur for me. I spoke with a lot of people who are close to me and Karen, relaying the story over and over. The more I shared, the stronger I felt. The more I relayed what I believed I heard from God, the more I was filled with faith. It was not like I was whipping myself into some false sense of emotional security. It was as if my spirit was preparing for a spiritual conflict that my mind could not really comprehend. This was going to be a battle. This was so much deeper and bigger than a sick dog. This was war!

SIX

WAR

A Brief Interuption

Sometimes, after a period of time passes, we can look back at a portion of our past and wonder why God did something the way He did it. Isaiah 55:8-9 tells us "For My thoughts are not your thoughts, Nor are your ways My ways," says The Lord. "For as the heavens are higher than the earth, so are My ways higher than your ways, and My thoughts than your thoughts." In this chapter I tell you about an oil which became a small part of our story. I am very aware of all the negative press surrounding the oil. It is tragic. Please understand that I feel I have been tasked with telling you this story in its entirety. I believe I am supposed to include every detail as it went down. Regardless of whether or not it turned out the way it was supposed to, all the details mattered at the time and therefore, they matter now. If your curiosity gets the best of you and you simply cannot read on, go research the story, or flip to the back of the book, to The Author's Final Notes, and read all I have written concerning it. However, I would like to encourage you to do that later. Take all of this as it happened to us chronologically and let it be what it is. To stop reading here only heaps tragedy upon tragedy. It is impossible to know all the details concerning the oil. All I can tell you is how it affected us and how it was a small detail in a large story; A minor ingredient in the recipe that displayed God's incredible Grace.

THE OIL

A few days earlier, on August 21, 2018 Karen called me from work and asked if I had seen her text. I had not. She told me she had heard the morning team on our Christian Radio Station, 91.5 talking about a Christian Bookstore in Dalton, GA where, apparently, there was a Bible that was leaking oil. I had heard of crazy things like this before and immediately chalked it up as some kind of gimmick, but I was interested enough that I told her I would look it up. I did. I was intrigued. It seemed quite supernatural and I, in my usual level of gullibility, thought it would be neat to go and see... maybe. Karen and I spoke briefly again about it at lunch and we agreed, we should go to Dalton sometime and see it for ourselves. That was it.

THE ELDERS PRAY

The day after the vet visit, August 29, I was reading my Bible about Jesus performing miracles. I was searching for strength in the recorded stories that would build my faith. Honestly, I think I was trying to find anything that helped me solidify what I believed. I needed some solidarity to hang this faith on because just 24 hours earlier I wasn't even sure God cared about dogs. I came across the scriptures that say, "If anyone needs healing, let them come to the church and have the elders pray over them." I called Travis and I led with that scripture. That is the way to manipulate your pastor by the way, lead with scripture! So, I told him what I had found and asked if I could bring Winston to the service that night. He agreed somewhat reluctantly I believe, and as far as I know, that was the first time a dog attended Wednesday night services (or any service) at Restoration Church.

During the day, I was speaking with my dad and something occurred to me that I had not thought of in weeks. We were talking about God still doing miracles and how I believed, somehow, that He was going to heal Winston. I suddenly remembered and therefore asked if he and Mom had heard about the Bible that was leaking oil, in North, GA. He had not, so, I showed him the video on YouTube. Dad got very excited and insisted that we call and ask if we could bring Winston up there the next day. Honestly, I thought he had lost his mind. I had no idea if what we were seeing on YouTube was even true. I told him I would think about it. I spoke with Karen, and she just so happened to have the next day off from work. My research led me to a bookstore in a small town in North Ga. I called the bookstore and explained what we wanted to do. I was told they would be leaving the next day for Alabama, however, if we were going to drive from Loganville, he would meet us there for a short time at 10 AM. He could not promise the Bible was going to be there, as he was not the owner, but he said they had some oil there at the store and they would pray with us over Winston. The plan was set.

That night, we sat in the back of the sanctuary and Winston was a perfect gentleman. At the end of the service, Travis told the congregation what I was doing there with my dog and invited anyone who wanted to stay and pray with us to do so. The response was overwhelming, and Travis prayed like I had never heard him pray. He didn't beat around the bush, he didn't ask for God's will to be done, he said, "We recognize you are sovereign Lord, but we want you to heal Winston…We aren't commanding you, Father, but asking in all the faith we have. Lord, heal Winston!"

OUR FIRST TRIP TO NORTH GA

At 7 a.m. on August 23, we loaded up and headed out to see what the Bible and the oil were all about. We were quite giddy but trying to be reserved about it all. I was still fasting, as my family members ate breakfast and drank coffee. It didn't even phase me as I had feared. I had been on a water-only fast since 12 pm on Tuesday, and I felt great. I believe God had miraculously sustained me, and I was not in the slightest bit hungry. I felt it was a confirmation that I was doing what I was supposed to be doing. We arrived in Dalton around 10:20 AM. Johnny, the man I had spoken with on the phone the day before, met us there and, to our surprise, Jerry, the owner of the Bible, was there and he had the Bible with him. I recognized both of them from the video.

It was a red leather Bible and was lying at the bottom of a plastic tub. There was nothing special about the plastic tub. In fact, I think it is a dog food container with a sealable lid. There were four or five inches of clear liquid in the tub in which the Bible was submerged. From the consistency of the liquid, it appeared to be a clear oil. Jerry reached into the tub and removed the Bible from the oil and showed it to us. The red dye in the leather was not being affected by the oil. The pages were not affected. The ink, even from the high-lighters used to mark scriptures was not affected. The binding was still intact, unaffected by the oil. It seemed amazing. At that time, the Bible had been leaking oil consistently and had been submerged in oil for nearly 19 months. At the time of this writing, it is still unaffected negatively by the oil and it has been 35 months. It has produced hundreds of gallons of oil to date and continues to do so. They feel they were instructed to give the oil away. They have freely given thousands of small glass vials of the oil away and have many stories of associated miracles.

I explained the whole situation about Winston to them. We gathered around Winston and laid our hands on him, they anointed him with some oil and one of them prayed for him. During the prayer, I felt as if God was saying, "Now, you have done all you can humanly, physically do. The rest is up to me." Afterward, Jerry gave us a bottle of oil and said it was just for Winston. He then proceeded to give us all our own bottles of oil.

When they handed Karen hers, however, the strangest thing happened. It was as if something slapped it out of her hand, and it hit the floor with a pop, and the glass bottle shattered. Oil poured out in a circle at her feet, and she looked like she was going to burst into tears. Karen is not the type to drop things, nor is she the type to burst into tears. It was very strange. They assured her it was no big deal, replaced her bottle, wiped up the oil and glass, and went on about their normal routine.

About 10 minutes later, a group of women came into the store and inquired about the Bible and oil. They were shown to the back where they gathered around the plastic tub which held the Bible and the oil it was producing. Jerry was speaking with them and they were all amazed. Suddenly, I heard one of them spontaneously begin to raise her voice in praise to God. I looked over and saw a lady standing on the spot where the oil had been spilled. The floor still looked wet and glossy beneath her exact location. She was not simply commenting about the oil, she was worshiping God in her own little church service! Now, I know, that might have happened no matter what… but no one else in the entire store had broken out in spontaneous worship!

After chatting with them briefly, we expressed our gratitude and left with Winston in tow, still hopping along on three legs. I didn't know what to do about fasting. I asked my dad, "Do you think I should just keep fasting until he walks again?" He reminded me of what God had said to me in the prayer, "You have done all you can do physically... the rest is up to Me." I had been on the fast for about 52 hours. I believed I was released to end my fast and suddenly I felt hungry. I turned to the rest of them and said, "Let's go have some Christian Chicken!"

SEVEN

BATTLES WON AND LOST

MY FRUSTRATIONS

I reached out to everyone I knew who prayed. In the following days several people I would consider to be prayer warriors, came by my house. Rico Ruiz came and laid his hands on Winston and prayed for him and us. I need to say, Rico was very reassuring but I could tell, he was very concerned about us as a family. That is the way he is. Filled with faith, Rico told me, "I am standing with you in faith, believing for God's miracle, but you need to know and recognize that God is sovereign. His will may be for Winston to die and you need to be prepared for that." I was. I just didn't believe that was God's will. Again, I could have been being hard headed. I continued to ask for prayer. My duck hunting friend, Corey Fenn, came by and prayed and cried with me over him. I was praying, but honestly, I wasn't even sure how to pray...I just kept thinking and praying "God, please heal him." I had faith but didn't know how to express it.

A week later I called on praying people from Facebook with this simple, direct post;

August 29, 2018
Facebook asks, "What's on your mind?" Ohh I have quite a lot on my mind. My main focus for the moment is a miracle. Google defines a miracle as; mir·a·cle mirək(ə)l/ noun   a surprising and welcome event that is not explicable by natural or scientific laws and is therefore considered to be the work of a divine agency.
(Here I re-counted the entire story of the Vet visit.)
I continued…
(I left the vet's office feeling filled with faith and confusion)… And then I was determined that I was going to see God's hand in a miracle on Winston. At first, my inclination said, "Do not tell just anybody about this, you don't want words of negativity being said over this situation!" But then, it came to me yesterday that this situation is "For someone" to see God's hand. Then without knowing about that feeling, my dad, Bob Rupard, texts me last night (which never happens at 10 pm) and says," Why would your dog have bone cancer if it were not for the Glory of God?" I thought that was a really weird way to put whatever it was he was trying to say… but then I got it.
Dad was reading last night and came across the story of Jesus healing a blind man, later the disciples asked him why the guy was blind in the first place… if he had sinned or his parents had sinned, which caused the blindness? Jesus answered by saying neither sinned to cause the blindness, but he was blind so that God would be glorified in the miracle of the day. Now, I cannot wrap my mind around all the "why's" and "what the hecks" involved in that but to me, it is simple for my situation. Winston had to get cancer for God to be revealed in a mighty way to someone.

And... frankly I don't care about negative words being spoken over the situation, those words are not MORE powerful than the Word of the Creator of the Universe!

Therefore, I ask you all to join with me in prayer for Winston's life. If you want to fast, there are some who are, and if you feel led to do so, I encourage that, if you DO NOT feel led to do so, then please don't.

James 5 says to anoint him with oil and lay hands on him and have the elders of the church pray for him. I know this is usually in reference to humans, but I feel like this is in good faith, and that is what we plan to do tonight.

For now, if you haven't met Winston, I have shared an incredible video of him when he was only 1 yr old. He is now 4 and is picking up 2 ducks at a time, fetching birds that fall 1000 yards away, and goes like a runaway freight train. He knows nothing but fun, fetch, run, and fills everyone around him with incredible joy.

Believe with me for God to perform a miracle. If you struggle with belief, then be like the man in Mark 9:14-19 when he said, "I believe! Help my unbelief!" If you ever pray, please pray for Winston's life.

There was a huge response to the post. A lot of people said they would be praying. Nothing changed. Winston kept limping in obvious pain and Heidi kept getting worse trying to urinate. I was praying over both of them, the same prayers with the same belief and with the same oil. No visible changes.

A few more days passed and Travis preached a sermon that had me questioning whether or not I had truly heard God's voice. I began to wonder if I had imagined it. I wondered if my mind was tricking me or maybe I was trying to simply manipulate God into healing him. One of the points of Travis' sermon was, "Often, there is a difference between what we WANT to be God's will and God's true will. Sometimes, that leaves us thinking we hear God's voice about something and because it lines up so well with what we want, it *must be* right! Oftentimes, that is, simply, not the case!"

Let me qualify this statement. This DOES NOT mean, if you think you hear God speak and it is something you *wanted to hear*, then it *cannot* be God. Obviously, He does not sit up in heaven, waiting to hear our desires, thinking, "Hmmm, now, how can I give them the opposite of that?" It simply means we should be careful not to project what we think is right or best or good, onto God. Often, His will looks different than we imagine it would.

I went home that day, wondering if I had truly heard God in the Vet's office or was it just what I wanted to hear. The agonizing problem was that I DID NOT hear, "I am going to heal Winston." I DID NOT hear, "Winston is not going to die." All I really heard was "If I cared enough about a man and his guitar, then I care enough about a man and his dog." Still, every day I knelt over him, as he lay in the floor, usually with tears streaming down my face, while holding his head in my hands, I begged God for his life. There were times I felt I may be wasting my time and energy, yet, somewhere deep inside of me, I felt like God was listening and He was going to spare him.

BEING OK WITH GOD'S WILL

This is a side note, but imperative. A number of years ago, after singing a song at church, I sat down in the pew and literally thought, "I nailed that!" I wondered pridefully how the people around me must have thought I could really sing. Seriously, I did that. It was a horrible moment of pride. The song was hard and I had really done it well. It was a Michael English song for pete's sake, give me a break! So, seriously, it was a moment of horrendous pride. Terrible, evil driven pride. And within WEEKS I began becoming hoarse, to the point I simply could not sing at all. It lasted for more than a year. I knew it was because of my pride. I knew that I had caused the problem, and I was sorry for it but it didn't change how hoarse I was. I confessed my sin over and over without change. Somewhere near a year later I was in the office of the church and I brought this up to my dear friend, Karen, who was in charge of the music. I think she may have asked about me singing again and I had to confess. I told her I didn't know if I would ever be able to sing again. I had been to the Dr about it and they were saying all kinds of different things but none of their medicinal efforts were changing my hoarseness. I told her I didn't know what to do. For brevity's sake, I will just say that she told me a story much like my own, in which she could not play the piano. She had to get to a point where she said if she never played the piano again, she would be "okay" if that is what God wanted. The proverbial "Not my will, but Thy will be done" and "It is well with my soul" and all of that. Well, it wasn't "well with my soul!" I *wasn't okay* with the idea of never singing again. The entire idea was quite foreign to me. However, over the following weeks it weighed on me very heavily. Finally, I gave in; One Sunday morning, at the alter, crying, I gave it up to Him and said, "if I never sing again, it is your will that I am most interested in. Give me a different gift or simply let me worship you in silence, but I am going to worship you none-the-less." Within WEEKS I could sing again. Yet, I should add, I have to be very careful with my voice or I can become hoarse in a moment and will not be able to sing. Invariably, before I have a time that I am supposed to be singing for a group or whatever, I suffer through some hoarseness. I truly think that there will always be that physical reminder that it is not in my own ability that I do anything, rather, it is in HIM that I operate and without HIM I can do nothing.

In the same fashion, I had come to grips that if Winston was to die, I was going to have to be satisfied, nay, joyful, in God's WILL, not my own. And I was working that out in my own soul, and once again, in my frustration, I turned to writing and to people. I have no idea why I do this. It makes me feel better to put pen to paper, so to speak, it makes me feel better to vent to the masses, I guess. I wrote on social media again. This time everything was a bit different.

September 3, 2018 Facebook Post;

So.[after] days of prayer. Days of Fasting. Anointing him with oil, having the elders of the church pray over him on the Alter of the church. Many people coming by and praying for him. Many, many more praying because of this post and other connections. It seems as if we all had any pull with The Father the Miracle would be old news by now. We'd be days past shaking our heads and saying, "Wow, God is so incredible! Look at that dog running around like there was never anything wrong." But, we aren't. We watch him limp or hop around helplessly, pitifully, painfully. The emotions are all over the place right now. Part of me has little patience for the Miracle to come. Then Travis Rutland preaches a sermon yesterday in which I felt like he could have excused the ENTIRE congregation prior to the service, came and sat down in front of me and said, God gave me this all for you. The fact is, I have not wanted to hear or think that "God's Will" might have been different than mine. I have not been "OK" if God's will meant that Winston suffered and died through agonizing bone cancer. But since yesterday morning I have had to learn to say that if God's will is for Winston to die, then, I will BE OK with that. For brevity's sake, I came to the conclusion that Abraham, when told to go and sacrifice Issac, had to come to grips with Issac's death, but somehow believed that God would miraculously save Issac's life. Guys, I know this is nowhere near as big a deal as Abraham and Issac, the Nation of Israel and all that, it's just a comparison. And I know Winston's life doesn't mean the same to the entire world as Issac's life. I'm keeping it real, but, to me, right now in this moment, his life means a lot to me, and I believe that means a lot to my God. Therefore, although I cannot see the evidence of a miracle, I am still believing that God will provide one. Ok with God's will, willing to give Winston up, if that is what God chooses for us, but believing that the Miracle is still waiting, still happening, still taking place, as I write.

EIGHT

THE WARRIOR

Monday afternoon, after the post had been out for the whole day, Karen and I were in the car going somewhere. (She probably remembers where and why, I do not.) She was driving. I scrolled through my phone on Facebook looking for answers to all life's problems. Suddenly, a message came across to me.

"God almighty, Your King and Saviour, has heard your prayer! ****It is in NO way, shape or form God's will for your dog to die!****BUT IT IS HIS WILL FOR THE CANCER TO DIE!! AND AT YOUR HANDS, BY YOUR COMMAND, CUT ITS UGLY HEAD OFF! YOU ARE A SON OF GOD WITH POWER!

Fasting and praying allows your spirit man(who is one with The Holy Spirit) to rise up and wage war and WIN! The key to victory for you is knowing God's will. 1 John 5:14,15. "If we pray ANYTHING according to God's will then we KNOW he hears us and if we know He hears us then we KNOW we

HAVE the petitions we asked of Him!"

Matt 10:8 "Heal the sick! Raise the dead! Cleanse the lepers! Cast out devils! Freely you received, freely give!

Don't forget, Matt 18:19 "if 2 of you agree as touching ANYTHING ON EARTH our Father in heaven will do it" John Jennings."

I said, "Karen, Listen to this message I just got from this dude." I read it out loud as we drove down the road.

"Who is that from?" she asked.

"Some dude named John Jennings. I feel like I should know him but I don't remember a John Jennings. He's a wild man! Dude is out there!"

"Tim!" It was the sound I get when clearly I should have known something that is as obvious as the nose on my face but my rotten memory has served me well again. "You know John Jennings....That's Anderson's dad!"

Of course it was John Jennings, Anderson's dad! You remember Anderson and his step father John. He is the young man who became my first prostaff member with Rais~A~Ruckus Game Calls. You met him in the first chapter as I rambled through how all of this started. Now you're beginning understand why I had to drag you through all of that history to tell you the whole story. You might be on the verge of seeing how God had been weaving an incredible web of disconnected strands.

The problem was, that was how I had him in my phone; "John, Anderson's dad", not "John Jennings." It made plenty of sense, as I mentioned before, John Jennings is one of those guys... the EXACT KIND OF GUY YOU WANT ON YOUR TEAM WHEN YOU'RE BATTLING CANCER!!

I made a phone call. I wanted to hear him in person. I asked if he would come and pray for Winston.

"When should I be there?" he responded.   .

We made the schedule and he showed up early. Grinning

from ear to ear as usual, John blasted in on our house with his normal enthusiasm and prayed and talked with us for 3 hours. During the time he was at our home, our mobile vet, Dr. A, came by to check on Heidi and talk with us about Winston.

Dr. A. wanted to take another sample from Heidi because, like Winston, Heidi wasn't showing any signs of improving. After gathering the samples she needed from Heidi, she and her husband came in and sat down in the floor to examine Winston. She had with her an emergency kit of sorts for when Winston's leg breaks. I say "when it breaks" because that was how it was explained to us.

She said, "The bone cancer eats away at the bone marrow. There is a tumor on the outside of the bone basically in a membrane that surrounds the bone as well. As you can see, on the x-ray, the bone wall is thinning and is considerably thin on one side. You need to keep him from putting much weight on the leg at any time. Put carpet runners throughout the house on the wood floors. The floors are slick and he will slip at some point while bouncing around on his three legs. He cannot ride in the car. He shouldn't be allowed to run at all. If he does, this is what you should expect to happen; the humerus will simply break from wearing thin. When it does, it will be a catastrophic break. Meaning, there will be nothing we can do for him. The bone will be too thin to be re-set. The cancer will be released into his bloodstream as well. This will be the time to make the decision to put him down. These medicines I am giving you will give him some comfort until which time you can get him to the vet or I can get here to put him down. One of them is a very strong sedative and the other is a large dose of pain medicine." She then explained to us about how to mix the shots and how to give an intramuscular injection. "He will be at rest in a few minutes after that and you will be able to handle him until it's done."

49

I knew it was the prudent thing to do. I believe in medicine. I believe in doctors. I believe that medical science is imperative and obviously God uses doctors (and vets) to help us in our times of need. I also know that medicine has its limits and clearly, we were up against a medical limit. The meds that were being sold to me were a preparation for all things expected by medical science. A preparation for the only outcome that medical science could consider. I believed the responsible thing to do was to buy the medications that were prescribed to him and give him those medicines. That is not a lack of faith in God's ability to heal. It was obvious that there was not an instantaneous healing. The meds were more for pain than anything. How cruel would I have been to refuse to medicate him through his pain simply because I believed God was going to heal him? There is a false idea among some people, who believe, if you have faith in God to heal, then, you should never go to the doctor or take medicine. They think it is "anti-faith" to put your trust in medicine, while you ask God for a miracle. I say, "Hogwash!" Even Jesus used outside influences during times of healing. I don't pretend to know all the answers as to *why* Jesus put mud on the eyes of the blind to heal them. Yet, He did. He had the blind man, whom I mentioned earlier, to wash in the pool of Siloam. In fact, throughout the Bible, in both Old and New Testaments, people and things were constantly being used to create miraculous circumstances. These circumstances were not because the miracles could not have been performed without the help of earthen fixtures or mankind. I believe the God who spoke into existence the universe could have spoken to the red sea and it would have parted before the children of Israel even arrived at its shores. Yet, God had Moses strike the waters with his staff. I believe that same God could speak to any of our sicknesses and they would have to leave. Yet, He still uses doctors to heal people. I do not think I am less faith-filled if I ask God to heal my head ache and take medicine in the same moment. I can pop an aspirin in full faith believing God will bring about the healing of my head. In Winston's case, I believe it was the responsible thing to do to be prepared for a worst case scenario. However, I was certain that Winston would never have need for the emergency shots. I believed God would heal him as I poured the oil on his leg and told the sickness to leave. On what, or whom, was my faith leaning? The oil? Jesus? My words? My faith? Yes. In all of it, I had faith. Ultimately, my faith is in Jesus and the power in His name. For, without Jesus, all the faith is useless, all the oil is simply ceremonial, all the words are wasted breath, but, *with Jesus,* all things are possible and all of these were graced with power. Yet, again, I digress.

Karen, John and I sat quietly listening to Dr. A. I sensed what was probably going through John's mind. I knew he did not accept what she was saying. Do not misinterpret this; He knew Winston had cancer. He simply did not believe it was going to advance the way she predicted. We all accepted, if we did nothing, her warnings would likely come to fruition. However, John believed, so vehemently, Jesus was going to alter the diagnosed outcome, he simply *knew* her prognosis was inaccurate. John is not the type of man who foolishly disregards the facts in some nonsensical stretch of religious belief. Conversely, he tells the scientific evidence it is simply misguided, not incorrect or nonexistent. He states the facts will not lead to the results predicted by historical or medical evidence. He stands on truth from scripture, founded in faith.

Romans 4:17 teaches us; "As it is written: 'I have made you a Father of many nations.' He is our Father in the sight of God, in whom he believed--the God who gives life to the dead and calls into being things that were not." The Apostle Paul was talking specifically about Abraham and his wife Sara, how her womb was old and had never been able to have children.

She was barren and way too old to have children, but God told Abraham that she would have a child. Take notice that the Bible does not say, "calls things that are as if they are not" The interpretation of this is God speaks *into existence*, things that are not. He did not say "Sara is not barren". He said, "Sara is going to have a child." For example, if I were sick. The doctor tells me, "Tim, you are sick." The Bible does not say, walk around denying the fact that I am sick. Is there pain? Do I have a sore throat? Do I feel terrible? Of course I do! Jesus didn't say to blind people, "Ohh, you're not really blind!" He said, "Your faith has healed you." Even when they didn't immediately feel healed and they still couldn't see. Sometimes they even had to go do something to fully receive their healing. Romans tells us to speak to the sickness and tell it what it IS! "It IS HEALED." Even when it doesn't feel healed. I call these "Faith Facts." Faith facts stand in the face of scientific or medical facts. That is the entire problem that faith creates. The scientific evidence says: The Earth is millions of years old and everything in it evolved. There is other evidence that flies in the face of that but the "faith facts" say it was all created by God, regardless of how old you think it is. The scientific facts say evolution directed single celled organisms to eventually become humans. Faith Facts say we were created human, from the beginning. Scientific facts say the universe happened by a random series of events. Faith facts stand on a belief that there was nothing "random" about the creation of the universe, at all. The scientific facts say cancer is there and cancer, in many cases, continues to grow and metastasize, and eventually, infects more and more parts of the body, until it takes over. In many cases it leads to death. That is what science says happens based on case after case, historical and medical evidence. The odds are hugely in favor of science until you introduce faith into the equation. Faith doesn't stick its head into the sand and simply refuse to see the facts. Faith does not decide that the facts are all incorrect and the diagnosis is bad. Faith looks at a situation, recognizing there are physical laws or rules in effect, and says, " there are other laws that are applicable that science doesn't typically take into consideration. Laws that are in place because the creator of the universe made them available to us. Laws that are often subject to the faith of the requester. Laws that require a person to stand up in the face of evidence and tell it that it is subject to a greater law, a greater power, and the greater power controls things that science and medicine cannot explain. It causes things to happen that will not fit into the mathematical or experimental boundaries of science…. "Inexplicable things."

Allow me to digress a little further. I think that God often employs medication and doctors to cure us. He undoubtedly granted us the understanding of medicine, hence I think we are meant to use it. I just believe where medication reaches its limitations, there we find a limitless Father who occasionally goes far beyond what science ever dreams possible. For some individuals, believing in God at all is a stretch. Accepting that He may indeed work a miracle in someone's life is something greater than they can wrap their mind around. That is all right. I believe God is great enough to handle the fact that some do not believe as of yet. As well, you may entirely refuse the notion of an evil power laboring to oppose God and all that is good. My Bible warns me he (satan) lurks about seeking whom he may devour, and he has come to steal, kill, and destroy. Consequently, his first impulse, when you muster any manner of faith, is to destroy it. This is the first way Satan attempts to breakdown your faith; He uses the observable, the visual. He uses the things you see, the scientific, the obvious situation at hand. He tells you that the doctors and what you can see are all that is real and true. He whispers to us that "faith" is a joke and is useless. He claims people with "so-called faith" are willfully blind and in denial. He states "faith" is for weak-minded people who need something to believe in. The biggest hole in all of that is when faith works. Now what? How does he explain that away? Our Bible teaches us, moreover, to "walk by faith, not by sight." That is not willfully blind nor is it simple. Walking by faith is very challenging. Walking by faith is deliberately believing in a higher authority than medicine and science even if you don't have personal experiences that can support it. Faith is not the negation of facts, faith is believing in THE truth. There is a difference between "the facts" and "truth." Faith recognizes that difference. Physicians can read the facts to you from their report. The TRUTH whispers, "read it in the Bible." The Bible explains in Isaiah 53 we are healed by his stripes. That is TRUTH. The truth then alters the facts. Truth + Faith, sways the facts.

On November 7th, 1997, I was traveling to work in the rain. I was driving a Geo Tracker with tires that should have been changed about 1000 miles earlier. I hit a patch of water and began to spin. I whirled uncontrollably off the right shoulder and made contact with the bank and proceeded to flip. The lady behind me informed me she lost count of the flips at 7. I should have perished in that accident. The Geo Tracker had the 2nd highest death rate, per accident, the previous year.[1] It is the third most deadly vehicle ever.[2] The car was demolished with the exception of the immediate area surrounding the driver's seat. Everything else was utterly destroyed. It came to rest on the driver's side. The window beside me didn't even break. I stepped out through the ripped rag-top unscathed. I felt I had experienced a miracle but it only began there. I was, of course, very sore from the accident. Everything hurt for a few days.

A couple of weeks later my back began to hurt. I don't think I truly associated the discomfort with the accident, at first, but in retrospect, I can see where it very probably, resulted from that. It seemed to get worse and worse. In late summer of 1998, I was beginning to miss days of work from the pain. It would get a little better only to return with a vengeance and be worse than ever. There were days I couldn't walk upright. The pain levels were about an 8 out of 10, if 10 was completely incapacitated from pain. I prayed and prayed. I begged God to heal me. I had the pastor lay hands on me and pray. I asked for prayer from others. By October, I hurt all the time. It hurt to sit, it hurt to stand, it hurt to lay down, it hurt all the time.

It was a Wednesday night and we were in small group Bible study. A guy named Ken was teaching. I was sitting in the chair, elbows propped on my knees because that was about the only way I could sit and find some level of relief. He was teaching on Isaiah 53. He read verse 5. I had heard this verse all of my life but that night I understood it differently. "But He was wounded for our transgressions, He was bruised for our iniquities. The chastisement for our peace was upon Him, and by His stripes, we are healed." Ken went on to speak about the particular tenses of the words "we were" and "we are". The very way this is written, clearly points out that the "healing" was something that was already done. *We are* healed. Not we are going to be or we can be or we might be. We are. It's done. As in, if the stripes happened, then so did the healing. And the stripes happened. John 19:1 says that Pilate had Jesus flogged. You can read tons of material about the flagellation of Christ and watch in graphic detail, the movie, The Passion of the Christ, if you so desire. Isaiah, hundreds of years earlier, prophesied about his scourging and wrote the words that through that scourging, we received healing. Ken said that night, "So, instead of asking, and begging, and whining to God about receiving healing, change your mind about how you receive it, begin to thank Him for the healing you have *already received*. Even if you don't see it in the natural, or feel it in your body, the healing has already taken place. It is a gift that has been bought for you and you don't realize it is there, so you don't think it exists. But it is there, so just start thanking Him for it." It was like a light came on for me and I genuinely went immediately into silent, personal prayer and said, "God, you know I don't feel it, but I accept it. I thank you for the healing in my back that is already there. I receive it. Thank you." I did not simply recite empty words. In faith, I received it and was genuinely thanking Him for what I just realized was there, waiting for me.

That was all I said. I opened my eyes, I did not change positions, I just sat there for the remainder of the Bible study. It lasted for a while longer, I am uncertain of the time span. As the study concluded, we prayed, were excused and everyone began to stand up. As usual, I proceeded to rise very slowly. It typically hurt terribly to stand, so, from habit, I moved gently to minimize significant pain. As I began to straighten my body I noticed I had no discomfort. It shocked me so much I didn't even tell anyone. I stood there in wonder as everyone was milling about, socializing. I sat back down in the chair. I stood back up rapidly. There was NO PAIN.

The next week I sat in my chair and recounted to the group what had happened to me. I stood and bent forward and touched my toes. I had not been able to do that for months. I was pain-free. I was healed. We ARE healed. As in, it already happened. As if the gift is lying under the tree and we need only to faithfully thank God for it, stroll in, pick it up, and claim it as ours.

In our case, or Winston's case, death was imminent according to all the vets. Let me recount here, the main vet sent the images to the head of the oncology department of veterinary sciences at the local university, then to my vet friend, Kieth Cox, in Flowery Branch Ga, then, I showed them to my mobile Vet. All 4 vets agreed on the diagnosis. All 4 vets suggested only one direction that bone cancer in dogs could go. Not a single vet gave us any hope other than aggressive progression and fatality. Science said, "You have weeks." Yet, I have digressed far enough.

In grace, John sat and listened intently with a professional and pleasant smile on his face. As the vet and her husband were leaving we cordially said our goodbyes and they drove away. John turned to me and said, "Your dog is not going to die. You are a son of The Most High God! Cancer has no place in your home, in your family, in your body or in the body of your dog. We are going to take authority that has already been given to you and tell the cancer to go to hell, where it came from and where it belongs!" Over the next hour or two John prayed and said so much to me and Karen that I couldn't begin to write it all. He bolstered my faith like it has never been bolstered. In the midst of it all, I can't remember whether he was praying when he said it or was talking to me, as it all is a bit of a blur, but he said something that struck me like lightening. In the midst of whatever he was saying, he said, "...in the name of Jesus, I command this cancer to dry up and die, by the power of the same spirit who raised Christ from the dead..." Let me repeat that; He said, "..By the power of the same spirit, that spirit who raised Christ from the dead..."

It shouldn't have struck me as something new. I know this because if Christ lives in me, then His spirit lives me, the Holy Spirit, The Spirit of God, and yes, He is the same spirit who actually raised Christ from the dead. Yet, it had never really struck me in that manner... within me, residing in and along side my spirit, is The Holy Spirit, the *same spirit* who actually raised Jesus Christ from the dead. And that spirit is empowered and empowers me to carry out what Jesus said we would do. His statement, those words, the entire idea or concept blew my mind in an instant. I suddenly realized that the releasing of power in my life was only restricted by my own doubt and fear. I had to be honest, as I have to be honest now, the words or thoughts, "power was only restricted by my own doubt" seem so inconsequential, so trifling. The truth is that those words are grossly inadequate to describe the size of the hurdle I was facing in my life. For me, it was like standing at the bottom of Everest, gazing upward into the clouds towards its masked peak, knowing that I had done all the things necessary to get there, the costs were paid, the travel was finished, all the preparations made, and "all that was left to do was simply climb the mountain."

When John said that and I took a moment to process it, I looked at him and repeated it. It felt like he was up at the mid-mountain camp, 10,000 feet in elevation higher than me and we were talking on the radio and he was saying, "Yes, just start walking Tim, come on up, the weather is great!" He saw the confusion, the excitement, and the fear in my eyes. He saw the reservations all over my face like I was saying, "That power may reside in *you, John,* but I think I missed that class."

"You're a son of the Most High God!" John almost yelled at me. It was at least the third time he had told me that. It was beginning to worm-hole its way through my thick skull. "I am a son of the Most High God…" I thought to myself.

I knew John was right. I knew the fact that God's Spirit, living in me, was the answer to all the questions. I knew that Jesus had told his disciples they would do even greater things than they had seen Him do. I knew I had experienced, to some degree, the miraculous power of God in my own life. I had seen Him do things that could not be explained. However, I could not see my way out of this one. I believed, or I wanted to believe completely. I felt God would answer our prayers and pleading. I felt in my heart, somehow, I would be telling the story of Winston to people who would suddenly believe there was a God who cared enough about us to even save our dogs and they would give their lives to Him. The problem was being fully committed to that faith. When John left that day, my faith was stronger than it had ever been. I was more convinced that God was going to heal Winston but the physical world screamed at me that I was an idiot, that I was blind to the truth and was just hearing "spiritual stuff" because that is what I wanted to hear. My entire core, my every cell wanted to believe every word that John spoke. I forced the belief into my mind and my heart followed. Or, maybe it was the other way around, I am not sure. All I knew for sure was this; I had been praying every single day, very often multiple times a day, *over* Winston. Now, *the way* I prayed was about to change. I would no longer be begging God for Winston's life, I was asking Him for His mercy and grace but I was also speaking directly *to the cancer* in the name of Jesus, informing it, by the power God had invested in me, it was no longer welcome. I was no longer on the sideline, urging the coach to do something about the game, I was His agent informing the opposition of how the game was going to go.

NINE

TEACHING TIMES

I have already relayed this story in Chapter 7, about my dad's morning devotion. But clearly, God was not finished teaching us through this text.

You remember..."Why would your dog have bone cancer if it were not for the Glory of God?"

It was a very strange text I received from him one morning. I sent back to dad that I wasn't sure about what he was saying. In a few seconds my phone was ringing. Dad began to explain to me that he had been studying the day before and read about a miracle that Jesus had performed. When the disciples had asked him about it later on, Jesus had explained that the man's sickness had not come as a result of sin but so that God would be glorified, in the moment. Dad went on to explain that he felt that through Winston's cancer and ultimate healing, God would be glorified which is why Winston must be going through this. He felt it was all to bring glory to The Father, and we would see it and be able to share it for His Glory. I believed dad was onto something and it helped me, in the moment, to justify my faith which seemed a little insane to my more analytical side. However, about the time I seemed to really be settling into this idea, Dad called back and told me he thought he may have been wrong. He was convinced he had been, in some form, attempting to manipulate God, trying to convince Him to heal Winston. He was telling God, "Look how this could glorify your name! Look at how many people we may be able to lead to you through this miracle." Suggesting to God that He perform a certain way so people would see the truth. In a way, I suppose he may have been trying to manipulate The Father. I was still hanging on to the first concept, God *would* be glorified through Winston's healing. That is scriptural, even though Dad felt convicted of doing what he did. I am still not convinced The Holy Spirit was convicting dad of manipulating God. I can't say with complete assurance that Dad wasn't convicting himself or even satan may have been lying to Dad, to make him doubt his discovery through his Bible study. Either of those ideas could have been very plausible. In any case, if God heals Winston, God WILL be glorified. And in my little bitty mind, that is a positive for everyone concerned, God included. Yet clearly, God does NOT need Winston to be healed to be glorified. He does not need to perform any particular miracle to prove anything to anyone. In fact, He commands us to glorify Him in ALL things, both good and bad. However, Jesus healed many people during His ministry whom He specifically instructed to tell no one how it happened. Remember, the basis of my dad's Bible study was the story about the blind man who was healed by Jesus and the disciples asked "Who sinned to cause this?" Jesus told them his condition was there so that God's name would be glorified through the healing. I believe in our limited way of understanding and in our western thinking minds, we do not interpret this scripture well. I believe many of us read it and work it out through logic. We are then left to think, "God struck this poor man blind (or allowed him to be struck blind) and left him that way, for however long he lived, until the moment he crossed paths with Jesus, just so He could be glorified through the man's healing. That seems oddly cruel. I truly believe what Jesus was saying was, "It was not sin that caused this, in fact, it doesn't matter *what* caused him to be blind, he was blind and he *was healed* so that God would be glorified." When I read Jesus' words throughout the Gospels, I read Him to be the kind of guy who would turn around and ask you, "What does it profit a man to wonder why this and why that? Why did he get sick? Why wasn't I born rich? Why did my friend have to die so young?" I think Jesus would say, "Why ask so many 'whys'? Just move forward in the direction I have given you and praise God for everything in your life! You have promises and untapped potential I have placed in your life. Go live in them and stop wondering "why" so much! It doesn't matter why, what matters is what you're going to do with it now." Whether someone is healed or not, changes nothing about the sovereign authority of God and His worthiness to be praised. I had to keep this in mind as I prayed over Winston and Heidi several times a day, anointing them with the oil, and telling the cancer to go, and telling Heidi's body to be healed and asking God for His grace and mercy, and praising Him for the outcomes.

GET UP AND LISTEN

I'm fifty-one years old. If you are around fifty then you understand that "sleeping in" is generally not an option. 3 a.m., 4 a.m., these are times that were reserved for hunting or perhaps fishing. Truthfully, I am a night owl, not so much of an early morning person. I get up when I need to, but I really don't get up early just to get up early. Nevertheless, for the last couple of years, every once in awhile I wake up around 3 or 4 and occasionally I feel God wants me to get up and pray. Let me state here, these have been moments that I have experienced incredible peace or personal revelation. It was always worth it to rise early. During this time, it was starting to be fairly regular, I would wake up and feel like I needed to get up and pray. Not necessarily about the dogs, but they usually tended to come up.

A few weeks into all of this, I woke up early. I didn't know how early it was, but it felt like 4:00. My eyes snapped open and I felt like I could hear God's whisper.

"Get up."

"Awe, c'mon Lord. It's very early, I'm very tired," I protested.

"Get up."

"Lord, seriously," I argued, "can't we do this at like 8? I am seriously tired."

"I don't want you to get up and pray, I want you to get up and listen." He not-so-patiently prodded.

Instantly, I was intrigued. Seriously, that was the first moment I knew it wasn't me or some strange aspect of my subconscious just "wanting" to get up and petition God for all the things I wanted Him to do.

"Listen?? Hmmm," I checked my watch. It was actually 5 a.m. "That's not so early anyway," I thought. "Alright, Lord. I'm coming, allow me get some clothes on."

I made my way into the kitchen and I began to quietly put on some coffee.

"Get water. I want you very clear." I Heard His voice in my soul.

"Okay…" I thought.

I made myself a glass of water although the coffee was beginning to trickle through the maker. I took a large swig of ice water and it cooled me as I swallowed. I sat down in my normal chair, placed the water on the table beside me and leaned back into the chair, causing the footrest to pop forward.

"Is that how you are going to approach your King?" I heard Him as clearly as if He was sitting across from me whispering loudly.

It stunned me. I sat for a second or two processing it. Both of these requests had never been made of me, nor had I ever heard of them from anyone else. I knew I was approaching something completely different than normal prayer time.

"Okay," I answered. I sat forward and the footrest slid back into place. I moved slowly, but deliberately, onto my knees on the rug in front of my chair. Leaning over I put my elbows on the floor, my head laid on my forearms. "Okay Lord, I am here."

"When the men you deem important (like Travis or Dr Mark Rutland or Jentzen Franklin) speak, you take notes. Don't you think you should take notes?" He spoke patiently at me. I felt it was more "at" me than "to" me.

Processing…..

"Okay…." I got up, dug out the small book into which I make notes, and returned to my position on my knees and elbows, pen in hand, the book opened to a blank page. "Okay, Lord, I am here." Then it happened.

My mind actually does not ever go blank. I have thoughts (and junk) racing every direction in my head. It's like a noisy buzz all the time. I think of work, family, relationships, church, and a list of things I need to do and lists of things I wish I could make happen. Literally, all the time, my mind buzzes. It would most probably be a psychotherapist's playground. However, in the split second, I stated, "I am here." My mind fell oddly silent. There was no chaos. There was no buzzing. There were no thoughts. Everything was absolutely quiet. All things were at complete peace, there was perfect serenity.

"Get Corey and Bob and go pray for D,"He began
I penned hurriedly while trying to process and listen.

He continued, "Winston and Heidi are hurdles and setbacks to prevent you from believing for D...."

I scribbled again hastily, trying to keep up.

"The oil is just something to help you believe," He spoke softly into my blank, silent mind. "Something to hang your faith on... but the faith is what heals you. You are as the woman who thought, 'if I can only touch his garment...' Touching His robe *was* the oil!" (in my thoughts, in an instant, I was reminded that in Luke, after the story of the woman touching Jesus' robe, the streets were lined with people who sought to simply touch His robe and be healed, and they were!) He went on, "Pray for this...   ...but I don't want you to tell anyone." (I *think* I interpreted that to be a guideline that meant "don't tell anyone about that for now, until I release you to do so.")

Either way, I refer back to the previous notation that Jesus healed people and then told people not to tell anyone about how it had happened. Apparently, God is still into keeping secrets for whatever reasons. He told me to pray a certain way and then told me not to tell anyone. I may be breaking the rule by just telling this! I don't know, I am in uncharted territory here. At least, for me, it is uncharted.

And as quickly as my mind had gone silent and peace had reigned in my soul for a few moments, the buzzing returned, my mind raced and thoughts filled my head. In my heart, I yelled out, "NO! We aren't done. Don't stop there! I have so many questions..." Radio silence. The voice that spoke to me like a hushed whisper, from somewhere inside of me, was as real as if it were speaking to me from someone sitting in the chair before me. That voice was gone. Tears welled up into my eyes. I wanted to pass the rest of my day in that peace. I wanted that feeling of being nearer to Him than I had ever been, to remain with me, but it slipped away. I needed to be able to question Him to clarify. I wanted to understand what His intentions were. I could hardly breathe. Tears streamed down my cheeks from needing more information and from exhilaration. God had genuinely spoken to me. It wasn't the first time I believed He had spoken to me, but it was unlike any other time He had spoken. Every time prior to this, I feel it was more like a correction. I had come to understand those experiences as "Mack-Truck in the intersection moments." At one moment I would be doing something and in the next, He was blowing my mind with some type of strong directive. This time was different. This time, I felt as if it was more like sharing, more like communication, like gentle instruction, while sharing of knowledge. These were not instructions that made any sense to me or things that I would have simply dreamed of, on my own. Although satan flooded the room with the temptation of doubt, it felt too genuine and made too little sense for it not to be authentic. I know, that sounds backwards. But if WE think things up, usually we can make sense of it. We see the plan beginning to end or at least the plan from beginning *towards* the end. We are logical in how we process things. At least, logical to our own way of thinking. But, when *He lays it out*, very often, it makes no sense in the beginning. That is where faith meets obedience and the miraculous becomes sensible and only on the backside of it all, can we make sense of any of it. That is why I say, "It made too little sense" NOT to be real. Let me explain why it made too *little* sense;

1. It had literally been weeks, maybe months, since I had even thought about D. Not a thought I tell you! She hadn't crossed my mind since Winston had been diagnosed. I was utterly consumed by his condition and she had completely and entirely slipped from my concerns. When I went back and read

what I had written, "I want you to take Bob and Corey and go pray for D".. I thought to myself, "Huh? D? What's SHE got to do with this? This isn't about D, this is about…well, ok."

2. As far as I was concerned, Winston was going to be healed, I was simply sure of that, and his healing had nothing to do with D. It had nothing to do with being a stumbling block or hurdle or a setback. Why would my own mind want to sabotage its own belief system? Heidi had zero to do with anything as far as I was concerned, she was just sick and should get better with medical treatment. To me, there was no connection between D and either of our dogs up until the very moment God connected them.

3. Hurtles and setbacks? Honestly, I wasn't even sure what that meant. My sensible mind wanted to reach for the idea that if Winston and Heidi were going to be setbacks and hurdles, that meant something negative would happen to them. It meant if Winston was going to "set me back," he would have to go through something catastrophic. In my mind, it meant that Winston would not get better, that he would get worse and that would shake me deeply. That wasn't even an option here. Winston and Heidi were going to be fine and that was that!

4. What does "touching His robe was the oil." even mean? As in, is there actually some genuine, true physical connection to the robe and the oil, or is that metaphorical? I understood the rest of it, there is nothing <u>magical</u> about the oil, even if it is <u>actually leaking</u> out of a Bible, with no scientific explanation. The oil is not greater or even equal to its creator. The healing still comes from Jesus. The power still comes from Jesus. The "healer" is still Jesus, and our faith in HIM is clearly what heals us. I have heard people talk about this many times. Sometimes,

we get things tangled up a bit. Do you need faith to be healed? If we look at scripture, we see that sometimes there was simply no faith at all, and people were healed. Lazarus was dead and his sisters fussed at Jesus. They said he should have been there sooner, that Lazarus' body had begun to decompose by the time Jesus arrived. There was no faith and Lazarus certainly did not exhibit faith, he was like…dead. Yet, he was raised to life. Then, there were those times Jesus said, "Your faith has made you whole." Clearly, in some circumstances, faith is a key element. But we dare not have faith in our ability to have faith, for it will fail you. We must place our faith in the one who remains constant, the healer, in Jesus, in God the Father. In times where the world, or science, or our peers, see the situation as hopeless, we must have faith in God, that He will do what He says He will do, and defy science, by healing us. God told me the oil is just oil. Yet, it is not *just oil*. Clear as mud right?

Let me try and make it more clear. By scientific definition, matter cannot be created, it can only be changed or modified. However, the molecular structure of paper cannot be modified to make oil. Especially, an amount of oil that continues to flow for 2 years without changing the molecular structure of the Bible and its paper. The Bible is not diminished, and the oil continues to flow. This oil is being <u>manufactured from nothing</u>. This defies science. It is, clearly, a gift from God. There are no ingredients being combined to make this happen. It is from the hand of God. Some may say, the owner of the Bible is pouring some kind of oil into the tub at night behind closed doors. It is what I believed at first, however, there are two different chemists who have tested the oil and cannot determine what it is. Secondly, the oil has power in it which also defies science. Story after story has emerged from people who have experienced this healing power. If I were to chalk those stories up as fabrications, I would be among many, I believe. However, I have experienced this power myself. Inexplicable situations have been associated with the oil in my own life. How do I explain these away? If seeing is believing, I have seen! What then? The oil is the robe and the robe is the oil because both were a "point of contact" with God/Jesus. The story in Luke 8:43-48 reveals a secret about this;

[43] And there was a woman who was having a discharge of blood for twelve years, and though she had spent all her living on physicians, she could not be healed by anyone. [44] She came up behind Him (Jesus) and touched the fringe of His garment, and immediately her discharge of blood ceased. [45] And Jesus said, "Who was it that touched me?" When all denied it, Peter said, "Master, the crowds surround you and are pressing in on you!" [46] But Jesus said, "Someone touched me, for I perceive that power has gone out from me." [47] And when the woman saw that she was not hidden, she came trembling, and falling down before Him declaring in the presence of all the people why she had touched Him, and how she had been immediately healed. [48] And He said to her, "Daughter, your faith has made you well; go in peace."

Jesus felt the power of the Spirit of God flow from Him when she made contact with the creator of the Universe. Although, she actually only made contact with His robe. Hence, "touching the robe was the oil." The same power that healed her is the same power which creates the oil that causes miraculous healing to happen. My only explanation is that it is an unexplained, powerful, point of contact with the creator of the universe.

5. Why would God tell me to pray a certain way? Why not just do to me or give to me what You WANT me to have? Why should I not tell anyone about it? If that happens in my life, everyone is going to KNOW about it. I could go on all day

here…. again, it made too little sense to NOT be real. None of these concepts are things my mind would have simply created.

So, there I was, with a list of things God had given me, awash in undeniable peace, yet, wondering what was going on in my life. I wanted to jump up and shout about what just happened, but I didn't know how much of it I was supposed to tell. I thought I might be losing my mind, but I was sure that I was not. I wanted to ask the people around me what they thought, but I didn't want people around me to think I was nuts. And, what did it all mean? What was I supposed to do with it? I had a few directives, therefore all I could think was to follow the instructions until I had more. That was my decision. I sat there, on the floor, and processed it, "Okay Tim, Let's roll!"

TEN

THE GOOD DOCTOR'S ADVICE

Attending a church where the lead pastor is the son of a world renowned evangelist, who has been the president of two major Christian Universities, and has been the lead pastor of several mega churches all over the U.S. has its benefits. Occasionally, Dr. Mark Rutland is at our church. In fact, he is there more than occasionally. He is there often. Being on staff at Restoration church gives me access to his wisdom, on a regular basis. Although, just attending the church is enough to gain some private conversation time with him, as he is very down to earth and is often sitting around before or after a service talking with people.

It was a Wednesday night before church and I happened to catch him relatively unoccupied.

"Dr. Rutland," I pried, "Is there any way I can have five minutes of your time?"

"Sure Tim, what's up?" he said, as we walked into the

foyer to gain a little privacy. I explained what I felt like God had said to me in my sitting room that morning. I explained it in the best detail I could recall, and I tried my best to use the words verbatim, as I had heard them.

"The first thing I am going to tell you, Tim, is the same thing I tell everyone who tells me they think they heard from God. Make sure you do not add to or take ANYTHING away from what you heard. So often, people hear something from God, add their own perspective or add words that fit better into what they had already perceived, and then start telling people that they had heard so and so from God, when clearly, that is NOT what God had actually said."

I assured Dr. Rutland, to the best of my ability, that what I told him was exactly what God had said.

"So," he continued, "I'm going to be 100 percent honest with you because you asked me to."

That made me nervous. But I agreed, stating that was the reason I came to him. I needed his honest opinion and wanted him to feel confident that he could be transparent.

"Okay, you should know, this is *only* my opinion. I am not saying I have some perfect translation or interpretation, but here goes...I have nothing to say about going to pray for the young lady... That seems perfectly in line with something God would say, in my opinion. Frankly, it sounds to me," he continued cautiously, "like Winston and Heidi may, in fact, die. God warned you of their demise to keep you from stumbling in your faith, for the young lady's healing. Maybe He knows that it would be a terrible blow to you if you lose them and wants you to not falter in your faith when you do. That may not be something you want to hear right now but you should be aware that a loving Father may simply want to give you a heads up to keep you from being devastated."

He peered at me to see if I was all right, I think, and then continued. "I would agree 100 percent about the oil, I am aware of it. Travis and I had heard of it when we were in Dalton, a few months ago, and I would say that what you believe you heard God say, about the oil, is absolutely sound."

That was relieving, at least. It seemed as if, so far, besides what he had told me about Winston dying, was at least confirming of how I felt. I looked patiently at him, waiting for him to continue.

When I told him the final thing I believed God had said to me, I explained it in greater detail. "God told me to pray for a specific spiritual gift. Then, told me not to tell anyone. I said, I may be breaking the rules by telling you this much, I am not sure!" I explained nothing further.

Dr. Rutland looked at me flatly and said, "He didn't say He would do anything! He just said for you to pray for it. Who knows *why* He would have asked you to pray for that? Remember, He didn't say He would heal Winston. He just said He cares for you."

The entire ordeal had been maddeningly frustrating; however, Dr. Mark was right. God didn't say "I am going to heal Winston." He said, "...I care enough about a man and his dog."

Dr. Rutland continued, "Tim, it sounds *to me* like your dogs are actually going to die, but God wants you to be prepared for that and wants you to remain steadfast in whatever He is asking you to do. The gift, whatever that may be, may or may not have anything to do with what He wants you to do. Just remember what I said: don't add to or take away from anything you felt like He said to you. What He said is sufficient. The EXACT words he said will come to be perfectly enough to fulfill whatever it is He is trying to convey to you. You do not have to infer anything to make it make sense... eventually it will, or it won't. But, what He says is enough, He doesn't need our help. You just have to be patient enough to see it through.

ELEVEN

SAME STUFF DIFFERENT DAY

I vacillated between being filled with faith and full of dread. I believed he was going to be healed but plainly, I could not *see* the evidence. I kept him on a regiment of Tylenol as well as an anti-inflammatory medication to help and reduce some discomfort. We were additionally giving him medication to promote bone growth utilized by people with osteoporosis. The vet explained it wouldn't cure cancer by any measure, but it may slow down the breaking down of the bone in his leg.

As the weeks continued to creep by, I would daily put my hands on Winston and Heidi. I would anoint them with the oil, I would pray with all the faith I could muster. I did my best to remember the encouraging revelation that within me is the same spirit that raised Jesus from the dead. Yet, the voice of dread and fear never ceased to haunt me, "..hurdles and setbacks to keep you from believing…" Everyday, I knelt over them, some days with tears flooding down the bridge of my nose. Other days I was strong as an oak, hoping to see a major change, wanting to be steadfast in my belief that God was going to miraculously heal my dogs. I talked with a lot of people about all of this, mostly people who were close to us. Some people were strong and faithful. Some were wavering, kindly trying to remind me that in God's sovereign will, the dogs could die. I think my attitude had them worried about me, if I lost both dogs. I think they felt that I would really crack up because I wouldn't speak of them dying. I wouldn't entertain that idea and wouldn't let anyone else really talk about that with me. I believe this worried the people around me. I am not one of those people who goes bananas over someone speaking negativity, nor do I believe a single negative or positive word out of our mouths can change the universe. In my honest opinion, I think often, we put too much pressure on ourselves and the people around us when we begin to demand that no one speak a word of negativity. I also think we may be placing too much faith in our own influence on the world around us. The truth is, God is working many things out, for many different people at the same time. I always think about that when I have an outdoor event, and I am praying that God keeps the rain away. The farmer next door may have been praying for months for rain, and here I am praying for sunshine. I do believe, however, there IS POWER in our words. Proverbs 18:21 tells us "Death and life are in the power of our tongue." I believe that when we say something over and over again we can help or hurt our own faith. If I walked around saying, "I believe God is going to heal Winston" to the people in my family, and then told people all day at work, "I don't know if God is going to heal Winston or not…" what am I doing to my own faith? The next morning I am going to have a hard time praying, aren't I? Notice, the Bible does not say, as it is often misquoted, "The power of life and death are in our tongue." It says your tongue has power, and that power can be as strong as life and death. This simply means that with your tongue, you can bring life to a situation, to a person, to their existence, or you can bring death to any of these. You can speak biblical truth to your children as they grow in your home and produce a confident, healthy thinking person, or you can speak death over them by insulting them, breaking down their spirit by constantly being impossible to please. A lying witness could literally cause a man to die on death row, while the truth being told in court could set an innocent man free. A single lie told in the circles of high school girls can destroy the reputation of an innocent girl and literally lead to her suicide. While a teacher, speaking good things into a young man's life could change his outlook and future dramatically. Life and death *reside in* the power that rests in the tongue. However, as in so many Bible verses, there is a primary application and a secondary application to its meaning. Verse 19 of the same chapter defines the primary application. It says a brother who is offended by your words is harder to win over than a strong city. We have surely seen this in our own lives. It continues to say that those contentions, (the hurt he is feeling) are like the bars of a castle. Meaning it keeps you at arms length, but it also traps him inside like a prison cell. However, the secondary application is found in Mark 11:23 where we are told to have faith in God, (not our words) but to *speak* to the mountain and then *believe it in our hearts,* and it shall be done. We cannot speak to some mountain in our life and then not believe it. Frankly, if you speak to the mountain and then go around saying to others that you don't know if it's really going to happen, then do you believe it in your heart? Now, here's the real question; Does your lack of belief negate the possibility of a miracle? Remember, many times Jesus did miracles for people that had no faith at all. However, notice that Jesus said in Mark, "Speak to the mountain and believe it in your *heart...* " Is there a difference between believing something in your heart and in your head? Is "believing in your heart" different than "Faith?" There may be some people that say I am splitting hairs on some of this, but I have to rationalize some of this in my head. How do we believe in our hearts? Some people would say, "I need to get my head around this, so I can believe it with my heart." I say, that is completely opposite of how God wants us to believe. Believe in your heart, through faith, watch the results and your head will follow. Your head believes what seems logical. You will never "wrap your head around" believing that cancer will simply dissolve and go away despite the medical evidence and images on the x-ray.

We all understand there are times when God performs miracles and times when He doesn't. I am ok with His sovereignty. I am all right with simply dismissing the question "Why heal this person, yet not the other person?" by stating that God is sovereign and He has His reasons and one day, we may understand them. There is a logical side of me, as there is in most of you, I am sure, that longs for answers about this. I wish I had them all. I do not. For now, allow me to finish "The Story."

I spoke scripture over our dogs. I spoke the words I had learned from my friend John Jennings. I spoke truth over them. Even, at times, when I had a hard time believing *in my head,* what my heart believed. I longed for unwavering faith. In some moments, I had faith. Other moments it was all I could do to push back and silence all my doubts. Karen worried about me. She is a logical thinker. She has boundaries and hard lines. Things are just the way they are with Karen. There is nothing wrong with that, at all. Those of us who have lines that are barely visible, need the hard line kind of people in our lives. For her, she wanted to believe what I believed, and I think she did, and still does, *in her heart,* but Karen is a person who likes to be prepared. She is an incredible hostess for these reasons, she thinks of everything. However, when you're faced with terminal cancer, "thinking of everything" is a dreadful plight. Being prepared means accepting that in most cases, the odds are against the miraculous and as much as she wanted to stand beside me, in the utmost faith, she felt that she needed to be personally prepared for losing Winston, as well as be prepared to deal with me, if we lost him. Because, to her, I was clearly not preparing for that.

OUR SECOND TRIP TO DALTON

Throughout this time, we anxiously waited for a miracle to happen. It was at the forefront of our minds, as we continued to try to maintain a normal life. Once again, as much as I was emotionally absorbed by all of this, I simply cannot fathom what it must be like to go through this with one of my children. Daily tasks remained basically the same for us. We had to get up and go to work, the dogs got fed in the morning and in the evening, and I attempted to make Winston as comfortable as possible by permitting him to lay on the couch in my office at home. There were days he remained there all day long, but I could see he was getting very tired of lying around. Occasionally, I would take him outdoors and hold him back, toss the retrieving toy about 6 feet away so he couldn't build up too much speed and allow him get it. We would do that about 6 times before his excitement level would frighten me to death, and I would have to make him stop. I couldn't prevent hearing the doctor's predictions about his leg snapping at any given moment and I feared it was going to happen while I was doing that. I couldn't bear to live with that thought, so we kept it to a minimum.

As I stated, we tried to live as normal as possible. The one thing that changed significantly around my house was our approach to prayer. I know my entire family was praying for Winston and Heidi, and there was less bickering and considerably more affection between us. Heidi was spending most of her time lying on her bed and Winston would hobble and hop around as much as we would let him, but it was easy to see his fatigue, in a short time. He still met us at the door, wagging his tail and panting, and he would still hop off into the yard as though he was running on three legs when we put them out to go to the bathroom. Occasionally, he would put some weight on his leg and limp, almost like he was trying to walk it off. Other times he wouldn't put any weight on it at all. The poor guy truly struggled to lift his leg and keep his balance while he was in obvious pain.

This consumed our lives. We were always talking about it with our friends, and I am sure they became tired of hearing about the dogs. However, we would get phone calls all the time asking about his status. A very special couple, Rico and Vikki, called very often, and through this time our friendship was deepening with them, rapidly. Rico is a bible thumpin', Spirit-filled Puerto Rican, with a heart the size of Texas. His little white, American, wife does all she can to keep up with him, as do we all! We began spending a lot of time with them. Sometime in September, they asked us about going to Dalton to see the Bible and get some of the oil. We agreed to go on a Friday morning. We all rode together in Rico's truck and left early that morning to make the store by 10:30 or 11:00. When we arrived Pastor Johnny was there and so was Jerry, the owner of the Bible. They received us as family and were disappointed we had not brought Winston with us. We talked for a while and Johnny finally called me off to the side to speak with me privately.

"It's crazy that you guys are here. I was praying just the other day and God brought Winston to my mind," he told me. Honestly, I was surprised because it had been a few months since we had been there, and this guy sees and talks to thousands of people from all over the world. Some random guy with a sick dog just doesn't seem to register high on the priority list, to me, considering all he is doing.

Johnny continued, "I had been reading about Jesus walking through the land, healing the people. The Bible said he *walked all through the land* and healed them, and I thought, 'God, why isn't Winston being healed instantly?' Then, I believe God told me, 'Winston is *walking out* his healing.' And that made sense to me, Tim. He's just walking it out like Jesus was walking through the land healing people, Winston just has to walk this out. He is walking out his healing." To be entirely honest, I thought Johnny was grasping at straws, but I wanted to receive what he was saying and allow God to work in whatever way He wanted. He certainly was doing his best to walk. I couldn't find anything un-Biblical with the concept, so I shook my head "yes" and told him I would believe on that. They gave us some more oil, while we were there, to give to others and to use. Johnny gave me another vial, specifically for the dogs, and we stayed and visited for a while with them. I was glad I had some oil to take by and give to D. I felt like it was time to go visit her and pray with her again, and now I had some oil I could take to her.

Sometimes, in life, seemingly disconnected moments, remain disconnected for a long time, until a light comes on and we notice something strange. We often find ourselves thinking, "Oh wow, if that had not happened, then this would never have happened" and so on. Oftentimes, we cannot see the whole picture of how things are connected, until years later. As I have written "The Story," I have found myself seeing God's amazing hand over the years, weaving it all together like a complicated tapestry of random pictures. The only way to see the connection throughout the tapestry is to take it all in, at one time, and only then, can the pictures tell the entire tale. If you only look at a few of the pictures, separately, you would never understand the entire plot. I remind the reader here to stay the course, because some of the details may seem disconnected. Some of these details may not come into clear focus, and we may not understand how they are connected for years after this is finished and, hopefully, read by thousands. You are going have to trust that I have heard from God, therefore, I must include whatever I have included. The next few "chapter-ets" may seem to be completely disconnected. I am trusting that somehow, I will be able to see their connectivity to the rest of this, someday. However, their timing and lack of "normalcy" would tell my spirit they are much more connected than we can imagine. So, humor me, while I drag you through my randomness.

COREY AND I VISIT D

I sent D a message and asked if a friend of mine and I could come by the shop and talk with her. She agreed so I called Corey and asked if he would meet me there. Nervously, he agreed. I knew I was putting him on the spot, but I also knew that God had performed a miracle in Corey and D needed to hear that God was still in that business. Corey, a year earlier, had been diagnosed with a brain tumor. Without going into the details, Corey poured himself out on the altar of God, praying for a miracle. The doctors were not super positive about the outcome of surgery but felt it was his best solution. We all prayed like we had never prayed before, for Corey and for his doctors. They did the surgery and when they went in, they found the tumor had never penetrated the membrane protecting his brain. It did not grow down into his brain like most do apparently, and basically, they opened his skull, pulled it out, closed him back up and in a couple days he went home and ate dinner, as if they had simply extracted a tooth. Everyone was amazed! Even the doctors were amazed. Did he require surgery? Yes. Was he miraculously healed like the stories you hear about people being prayed for and the next thing you know the doctors cannot find anything anymore? No. Was he healed and not touched by cancer and do we believe it was a miracle? I believe so. Corey stands on it to be a fact. Corey told his story to D. We asked if we could pray for her and she timidly said we could. I asked Corey to pray. I gave the oil to her and explained the story surrounding it as best I could. She thanked me and thanked Corey for coming by and we left. No singing angels, no bright lights, nothing spectacular happened. Yet, I believe D is being healed.

TWELVE

THE PROPHECY

In October every year, there is a pastor's conference in Puerto Rico. I have been associated with the church that hosts the conference for years and have attended the conference a number of times. I speak semi-fluent Spanish but I'll never forget, the first time I attended the conference. The entire time I was there, I only understood four words during any of the conference meetings. Those words were, "Hermano Tim, de Georgia!" (Brother Tim from Georgia) I would smile and wave the little hand-twisting wave of a celebrity riding in a car through a crowd, nod my head as if I knew what was being said about me, and slump back into my mind numbing state of total ignorance. Puerto Rican Spanish is NOT like Spanish... it's something else... but it's not the Spanish like I had learned! I understand they throw some Spanish in there for good measure, and most throw some English in there as well, just to really confuse you. They also speak at a rate that is not humanly possible to understand. They drop letters from all their words. They use all kinds of slang. They add sounds that are not in any other Spanish speaking dialect. They combine words to make their sentences shorter. It is more aptly named, " 'Rican Spanglish." It's Spanish but it's not Spanish! These days, after much more experience, I catch enough to get the gist of what is being said, and I do pretty well in basic conversation with my "hermanos de Puerto Rico," and I love spending time with my Puerto Rican family! So, in October, 2018, Rico and Vikki, and Karen and I went to the pastor's conference together.

Karen had learned in September of a particular need for little girls' dresses for Christmas. There was a lady, in the church in P.R. we were visiting, who was going on a mission trip of her own, to the Dominican Republic, at Christmas time. She wanted to take dresses to the little girls in the D.R. Karen had started a campaign at our home church to collect dresses, for our friend to take with her. She collected a LOT of dresses, and two pairs of shoes. We needed to take them with us to P.R. in one luggage bag which we could give to our friend to take with her to the D.R. The bag could weigh a maximum of 50 lbs. We received, as a donation, a piece of luggage that was large enough to hold all the dresses, and just so happened to be the lightest luggage made to date. Unpacked, this huge suit case only weighed 2.5 lbs! Therefore, it would allow us to take more dresses. A week or so before we left, Karen stayed up one night to pack all the dresses into the bag. Amazingly, they all fit. The two pair of shoes remained unpacked, sitting in our dining room. She struggled with whether or not to take them. They were extra weight and honestly, she didn't think they would fit. The suit case was FULL! She felt as if it would be overweight already. Plus, she wasn't supposed to bring shoes. She felt she was supposed to be bringing dresses.

"Take the shoes." She thought God told her.

"This is ridiculous." Karen argued. She walked by the suit case for several days resisting.

"Take the Shoes!" She would hear, every time she walked by or thought about it. Finally, she conceded with frustration and crammed the shoes into the bag, feeling certain she would have to remove them at the airport because of the weight limit. This was a large suitcase stuffed full of dresses and two pairs of shoes. The zippers were straining and it bulged everywhere. In my opinion, there was no way it would pass the weight check.

At the airport, Karen plopped the bag on the scale knowing what was coming. Click, click, click... the scale settled in... 49.5 lbs. We all smiled at each other in amazement.

"Hmmm, I wonder what those shoes have to do with this trip." Karen thought.

We had a few days of much needed R&R. Then, on Sunday, we drove down to the main service in Ponce, about 2.5 hours south of where we were staying in Fajardo. The church was small. Much too small for the crowd that was there. However, they had saved 4 seats right up front for us. They supplied a personal interpreter for Karen, and I was going to do my best to catch what was being spoken. Rico interpreted quietly for Vikki and the service started. The guest preacher finally took the platform and wow did that guy preach. Then, in the middle of the sermon, things took a little bit of a strange turn. He was talking about walking out what God had called for you to do. Walking it out with pleasure and excitement. I could identify with the sermon pretty well. It was the same idea I preached using Winston as an example many times before. Suddenly, he stopped preaching, pointed at Karen and me and asked the pastor of the church who we were. I heard Karen's interpreter trying to stammer through what was going on. The pastor answered him, explaining we were "pastors" from the US and said we were more like missionaries. (I am the Missions Pastor at our church so that was about as accurate as could be explained, in the time frame given.) He looked at us and began explaining that he could see money pouring through my hands. Thousands, maybe millions, of dollars pouring through my hands. Then, he went back to preaching. Just like that. I didn't hear much after that moment. I had no idea how to begin to process what he said. It made no sense to me. After he was finished preaching, he asked all the pastors and their wives to come to the front. We stayed in our seats assuming it was for the pastors of all the churches represented there in P.R. The head pastor came over to us and urged us to come to the front and as I stepped up to go, Karen hesitated, shaking her head, "no" and said, "I am not a pastor." The Lead Pastor Miguel explained to her that she was as much a pastor as he was and she needed to come to the front. She followed me to the front, sheepishly. The guest preacher began laying his hands on the pastors and their wives and praying over them. They all seemed to respond normally and from what I could hear and understand, the prayers were basically generic. He prayed for them to be blessed and protected. He prayed for their finances and for their congregations. He then came to me, laid his hands on my head and prayed the same kind of generic prayer. "Father, bless him, keep him in your will, protect him, etc." He finished praying over me, placed his hands on Karen's head, closed his eyes, furrowed his brow and stood there silently. I watched him closely. Karen looked up at him. I could feel her discomfort. She is not a "touchy-feely" kind of person. She would rather have someone keep their distance than come up and give her hugs or put their hands on her. He opened his eyes and instead of praying, he spoke to her. I tried to hear it all but his Spanish was so fast. The interpreter had come with us, for Karen's sake and he talked quietly into Karen's ear as the preacher spoke what he was seeing. "I see you standing somewhere. Children are running to you. Lots and lots of children. They are all running to you. You are giving them shoes, thousands of pairs of shoes." I understood that part and every hair on my body stood at attention. I saw Karen's eyes widen and fill with tears as the interpreter explained what had been said. Shoes. It was some light on the struggle she had with God, over those shoes. There were *tons* of unanswered questions and even more doubts as to how that could possibly come to pass. But in that moment, standing there in a tiny church in Puerto Rico, being prophesied over by a preacher who had no idea who we were, nor had he any idea about the dresses or the shoes, or what we had been going through, it all felt like God was saying, "I am going to give you a glimpse of what I am doing, and I want you to know I am in charge of it all and I have you and your life in mind."

THIRTEEN

ALL THINGS NORMAL EXCEPT EVERYTHING

My Christian walk (I think) has been pretty normal for most of my life. I have my issues with which I struggle. I spent most of my career life in construction so, I struggled with my language, for one. In that industry, as it is in many, most people curse...a lot. It was something that I truly hated about myself; Regardless of how spiritual I became, or how much I prayed or studied, or how much I taught or sang, outside of church and with the exception of when I was in the presence of my mother, I cursed like a sailor. I had what I thought was a normal kind of prayer life. I prayed most days, sometimes more, sometimes less. My personal study time has always had an ebb and flow to it. I would get in the habit of studying or reading a personal devotion type of book, and then I would fall out of the habit. I always wanted to do more, be better, act more "saintly" I suppose, but there was always something in my life that would take precedence, and I would lose my momentum.

When this thing took place with Winston, my sister challenged me right off the bat, to show God how serious I was, by fasting. My daily prayer habits changed dramatically. Isn't that always the case though? We find ourselves in a great time of need and suddenly we are like BFF's with God. My Pastor, Travis, says often, "There are no atheists in foxholes." And it's true. When we need Him the most, we can be prayer warriors, but when everything is smooth sailing we forget to even say "Thank you."

I use the words "prayer habits" because what I believe I lacked most in my life, was the habit of communicating with God, throughout the day, about everything. 1 Thessalonians 5:17 tells us to pray without ceasing. Colossians 4:2 says, "Devote yourselves to prayer, keeping alert in it with an attitude of thanksgiving." Prior to this time in my life these ideas seemed somewhat foreign to me. How do you go through your day, doing your normal activities and jobs and "pray without ceasing?" That seemed, to me, like something reserved for monks. However, it became more and more real to me, that even while performing the most mundane tasks, a prayer was always just a breath away. It suddenly seemed as if His presence constantly accompanied me, and I just conversed with Him all day long. The more I was in this "attitude of prayer," the more I began feeling like He was talking back. I began "hearing God" about many things. Even as I write this, it makes me feel like the guy in the movie, Close Encounters of the 3rd Kind. No, I didn't start building clay mountains in my living room, though, there have been moments when, I am sure, my friends and family have thought I had slipped over the edge of sanity mountain, into a place reserved for people wearing tinfoil hats. I was beginning to really wonder about myself and my sanity. Part of me questioned whether or not I was truly hearing from God, or was I just wanting to hear from Him so much, I had become a little delusional. I am analytical like that. I don't have any problem with an ultra-spiritual God who operates in the supernatural. I may be freaked out a little by something supernatural, but I believe that He is perfectly capable of doing anything He wants. I learned a long time ago, "Don't put God in a box." However, I never want to be associated with a circumstance where a human, especially myself, manufactures something that only appears spiritual, for whatever reason. In the world we live in, I believe there have been many well-meaning Christians who have done this and in my opinion, there are few deceptions more evil than a "manufactured spiritual experience." With that in mind, I had been hoping for God to give me some confirmation that I wasn't losing my mind. I wanted to know I was hearing from Him and not just dreaming up things and calling them "His voice."

Sunday morning started just like a normal Sunday morning. During praise and worship, around the beginning of the second song, I sat down in my chair and began to pray privately. The worship was exceptional that day, but I just felt like worshiping and praying quietly. I felt the hands of a person, behind me, rest on my shoulders. She began to pray. I realized it was Sylvia, the head of the prayer team. I couldn't hear what she was praying. Then, she leaned over so I could hear her and said, "You are walking in Jesus' footsteps in your ministry. He has plans for you to do great things, continue in His footsteps. The ministry He has given you is yours. Walk in it, He is with you." I sat there wondering what it all meant. My pessimistic side rose to the surface, and I thought, "Am I going to die? Is that what she is talking about being on His path and in His footsteps?" It made me wonder what all of this was about and what I was supposed to be doing. Just to be clear, Karen and I spoke very little, to people at our church, about all of these things that were happening in our lives. We have very specific people we talk to regularly, but we do not make the details of our lives well known, to everyone. Sylvia would not have known anything about the prophecy in Puerto Rico, nor any of my personal struggles or concerns. She would not have known I was searching for answers about God speaking to me.

There is a story in the Old Testament about a man named Gideon. To be brief, Gideon was the low man on the totem pole of his clan. His clan or tribe was the lowest order of the tribes of Israel. At this time the Israelites were being tormented, hunted down, and killed by the Midianites. The book of Judges records that Gideon, being deathly afraid to show himself out in the open, was inside a wine press. It reads as if he were down inside a cavern-like structure, hiding while threshing wheat. Wheat threshing is best done out in the open air where the wind can blow away the chaff. In a wine press of any sort, there is little-to-no wind. He was there trying to get some grain to make bread for his family without being seen by the Midianites. An angel appeared to him and addressed him as a "Mighty man of Valor." He argued with the angel stating he was far from a mighty man of valor, but the angel told him that he had been chosen to lead an army of Israelites to defeat the Midianites. Gideon basically runs the angel through a vetting process to make sure he is really an angel, regardless of the fact he simply appeared from nowhere inside the wine press and knew him. Later in the story, he thinks he hears from God again and asks Him to prove that it is Him. He said to God, "if this is really what you want, then I am going to lay this blanket out on the ground tonight, and I want you to let the dew fall all around it on the ground but keep the blanket completely dry. The next morning, that is exactly what happened. However, still, in doubt, Gideon challenges God again, to do the opposite thing. "Keep the ground dry tonight, but let the dew fall only on the blanket." I guess the first night wasn't quite enough proof that God was actually telling him what to do. Often, I look at that story and think, "Man, how much evidence did you really need?" But, then I catch myself doing the same thing. I experience something virtually impossible, clearly seeing God's hand in it, and still, I need more evidence of His presence. Even after Sylvia prayed over me out of the blue, and told me what God had put in her spirit, I still questioned my place, His will, His desire to use me, and my abilities. A few weeks later He showed me more.

About the same time in the service, around the second song, I felt like God was telling me to go forward and say something. This had happened once or twice in five years but I didn't like to do this sort of thing. This time, I sat and tried to listen, to know what God had for me to say and He said, "Go up there and tell Travis you have something to say... I will tell you what to say when you get there."

"Ohhh no... that's not how this is gonna work, Lord. You gotta give me SOMETHING before I step out like that... I can't just go up there without any idea of what I am supposed to say." I argued. I sat down in my chair defiantly and leaned forward, elbows on my knees, to pray and argue and hide like Gideon. "I have faith, but not that kind of faith... clearly you have tapped the wrong guy." It seemed like an all-out war in my head. All I could hear was the constant sound without a sound, the statement, "Go to the front, I have something for you to say." But it wasn't like being said over and over. It had been said, and then it lay there in my mind as if it was still being said, beginning to end without being repeated. It was just there, a constant existence. By far, it was one of the strangest ways I have heard God's prompting. Much like a question, waiting, demanding to be answered while the questioner just sits there staring at you. I know how crazy that sounds.

I began to sweat and my heart pounded. My hands got cold and clammy and Karen reached for my hand, as she could tell I was disturbed. She felt the temperature of my hands and the sweat on my palms and reached up to my forehead. I looked at her and she asked if I was okay. The frustration must have been very evident as I shook my head yes. She furrowed her brow and asked if I was sure. I resumed praying and arguing. The song was beginning to end and I knew the window was closing for me to be obedient. It wasn't going to happen in obedience. I wasn't even lifting my head without some sort of words from God. Faith is hard enough, blind faith where I am way out on a limb, with no safety net and no idea what I am doing there, that kind of faith was going to have to be the faith of another guy. "I can make a total fool of myself without the help of the Pastor and the congregation and some yet-existent word from the Lord," I argued to The Father. Yet, the request simply remained "there."

The song ended and Travis, as he usually does in our service, stepped up to the platform and turned to address the crowd. I didn't even look up.

"I don't usually do this," Travis started, "I just feel that God has something for someone to say. I feel like God is speaking to someone and giving them a message for the church, and I do not want to go further into the service without giving the person the opportunity to do what, clearly, they are supposed to do."

My blood ran cold. I knew that it was directed at me. I knew God was calling me out. The pressure grew by the instant, and I wanted to crawl under the seat.

Suddenly, after a long, uncomfortable pause, Silvia, the same lady who prayed over me, spoke up. She spoke clearly and loudly. "I am here with you, I love you, I have called you and I will go with you…. You come here for my Grace and Mercy and I give it to you…. I will put the words in your mouth because I AM the Word! … I am your healer…I am with you."

As far as I was concerned her message was directly for me. Although it saved me from going down to the front and speaking at the moment, it was an encouragement for me to step out and walk in faith. And God had not finished calling on me. He wasn't letting me off the hook that easy.

Travis spoke about the prophet Elijah and his altar, in his sermon. At the end of the sermon, during the altar call, God's voice came to me again. "Move. I have something for you to say."

I had no idea what I was about to do or say, I just knew beyond a shadow of a doubt, that I was supposed to go to the front. When I got there Travis was on his knees at the altar praying. I put my arm around his shoulder and prayed for him for a moment. When I was finished, I leaned over and told him I thought I had something I was supposed to say to the church. He looked at me and whispered, "I'm glad you came down here, I thought I was going to have to come back there and find you! God told me you had something to say, you were who I was talking about earlier…but I don't know what happened earlier. Also, please just close the service in prayer as well."

My mind was spinning and I REALLY didn't want to close the service in prayer. As Travis got up to the platform again to tell the congregation what had just happened, I prayed feverishly for God to tell me what to say and how I should pray to close the service. "Read Elijah's prayer to close the service." I heard it as clear as a bell. "Now speak." Travis called me to the platform and I took a microphone. I admitted my reluctance to speak from earlier and told them God had fussed at me about sitting in my seat. I thanked Sylvia for saving me earlier in the service and I realize now, no one understood what I was talking about. I moved on to reiterate what Travis had been talking about with Elijah and the altar, and God gave me an analogy about the weeds in our front flower bed. Karen had said, just days before, that she was going to rip it all out and kill everything in it so she could start over, and that was what God wanted to do in our lives. Rip out all the bad stuff and replace it with something beautiful. I kept hearing the word "forgiveness" so I said, "If you are harboring un-forgiveness in your life, it is like a poison you are drinking, hoping it hurts someone else. You need to let God rip that out." Then, I spoke directly to Travis about the Spirit of the Church and how God was going to unleash power on our church in the not-too-distant future. I got emotional and finished, handed the microphone back to him, and left the stage.

I had FORGOTTEN TO CLOSE THE SERVICE! Travis, being a professional, stepped to the platform and said, "I want to close with reading the Prayer of Elijah over our church." It was THE EXACT same thing God had told me to do! I stood there, just off to the side, and realized I had forgotten to do it but God clearly wanted that done. Travis looked down at the Bible to read it and fell silent. He covered his face with both hands trying to compose himself. In five years, I had not seen him so incapacitated. I stepped back to the platform and told him I would read Elijah's prayer. He slumped to the floor beside the podium, on his knees and face, in deep prayer as I read from 1 Kings 18:36. "At the time for the evening sacrifice, the prophet Elijah went near the altar. 'Lord God of Abraham, Isaac, and Israel, let it be known that you are the God in Israel and that I am your servant, and that I have done all these things at your word. Hear me oh God! Hear me, that these people will know that you are Lord God and that you have turned their heart back again.' "

A long time ago, I had a good friend who was a pastor. He invited me to speak to his church and I, being very young and inexperienced, asked for his advice on preparing a sermon. He said, "After you have prayed and studied and jotted down the notes and prepared an outline, you will know, to some extent, what you want to say. Then, ask yourself, 'So what? What is the point of it all? What am I trying to get across to my listeners in all of this?" I mention that now because you may have read through the last few portions of this book and you may be asking yourself, "What's the point of all of this? It seems as though Tim has taken some strange turn that has nothing to do with his dog or cancer." Therefore, allow me to explain myself. I believe God uses small things to push us along the path. I may never have been able to believe that I was hearing from God, about Winston, if He had not moved miraculously in a service. But while I was "walking out my faith" with Winston, it was vital to know that He really WAS in the middle of it all. I could have easily convinced myself that God wasn't speaking, there was no healing taking place, and that I had dreamed it all up, grasping at some kind of hope that something positive was going to happen. I am not writing this portion of the book for the reader to feel like I am something special or to boast. I am writing it for the same reason I believe God gave us the oil, for something "tangible for you to hang your faith on." I am writing it to strengthen your faith.   You do not have to believe any of it. That doesn't change whether or not it is true. You can reason it away as a coincidence. Although the service I just wrote about is recorded and on the church website somewhere. Yet, as I continue, you may see there was a lot of "coincidence" that had to happen, in a short amount of time. You may spin it all as some cosmic sense of positive thinking that causes people to act a certain way and for good things to happen. Do what you must. I write this to help you believe there is a God who cares, a God who performs miracles, and a God who sees you. I write this in full knowledge of the fact, there are going to be people who read this and have different results. That is another thing that satan uses to tear us down. He says, "Okay, you have faith and all of that, big deal! It is faith in a God who is busy with the rest of the world doing His important God stuff. He is not involved in the trivial aspects of your life. He will not do it like you think He will, and when He doesn't you're going to look like a total fool!" Matthew 10:29 tells us that God sees even the tiniest sparrow and is concerned about its life.

HAVE FAITH

How many times do you think that statement has been made? It almost seems ridiculous to write it. Have Faith. The epitome of cliche. At the same time, it is likely one of the most powerful statements in the universe. We live in a world in which it seems silly of me to write about the definition of faith but, I must. Hebrews 11:1 says "Faith is the substance for things hoped for, the evidence of things unseen." That's just fancy, isn't it? Let's break that down a bit. "The substance of things hoped for" can be re-stated like "stubborn belief that the things we hope will happen, will actually come to pass" and "the evidence of things unseen" means "the conviction within us that there are "things" or "entities, actual beings" that we cannot see. i.e. God the Father, Jesus His Son, The Holy Spirit and angels, etc. So, Faith is defined pretty basically in that statement. There is a human dilemma with this though. James addresses it but it makes us feel lousy. James 1:6-8: "But let him ask in faith, nothing wavering. For he that wavereth is like a wave of the sea driven with the wind and tossed. For let not that man think that he shall receive anything of the Lord" Over the years I've really struggled with this. Who doesn't "wavereth?"

I am an analytical kind of guy. I always want to know the "hows" and "whys". As a young adult, there was always this nagging question in the back of my mind that asked, "What if all of this is wrong? What if when we die we just turn back to dirt and all my beliefs about God are false? What if I am wasting my time and energy because there really is nothing there?" I would argue those questions back into their place in the dark recesses of my mind. I would rationalize through them with Pascal's Wager. "It is better to believe and be wrong than to not believe and be wrong!" However, there were times when I truly struggled with the heaviest word in the book of faith. Doubt.

While faith can lift us to untold heights, doubt is like an anchor that plunges us to the depths of the sea. That is why the verse in James makes us feel so inadequate. Many of us deal with doubt. It is sneaky. It is like a fog that creeps up on us. At first, it just begins to obscure our view but, before you know it, it has left everything soaking wet and you can't see but a few feet ahead of you. Doubt can leave us wandering in the dark and there's no part of life it doesn't affect. It is the enemy of faith and to allow them both to have a place on the battlefield of the mind is treacherous to your walk in Christ.

Somewhere around 2001, I was involved in a church (the same church as the chapter 7 story about being hoarse) that performed a huge Easter presentation. I sang on the praise team at that church and was involved in leadership. Every year we would do this presentation and that same dear friend, Karen, asked me to sing a song about miracles. It was a beautiful song that describes several miracles that Jesus did throughout His ministry. I thoroughly enjoyed singing it. We would perform this two weekends in a row, on Friday and Saturday nights.

On one of the Saturdays we were doing this, I woke up and the spring-time allergies had come on in full force! I was completely hoarse and could barely even speak. It was crazy. Usually, that kind of thing happens slowly, but not this time. I woke up and couldn't talk. I did everything I knew to do to restore my voice and finally that afternoon I arrived at the church and went to Karen and shocked her by whispering, "I cannot sing tonight!" She didn't panic. There was an incredibly talented young lady on our praise team who had the uncanny ability to know everyone's songs, lyrics, parts, etc. It is a talent that I am completely incapable of even understanding. While I have always struggled with my own part and remembering words, she could, in an instant, step into any part, in any musical, and not only do someone else's song for them but very likely do it better than they could! Her name is Brooke Gouge and she is a fantastic vocalist. Karen told me to go tell Brooke that she would be standing in for me that night and she needed to go over the song. I did as instructed. Quickly, it spread that I would not be singing the miracles song that night. I didn't get dressed in costume, and I planned to be in the crowd for the night.

"Tim!" a familiar voice sharply spoke to me. It was a dear friend of mine, Rod Johnson who attended church there. Rod was a force of nature both physically and spiritually. As a probation officer in the Walton County area, his name struck fear in the hearts of the men and women who violated their parole. When Rod came to see you, it was best to be on the right side of things! I am also sure that the demonic world knows his name in the same manner. He's a spiritual giant in my opinion and the kind of guy you want on your side in a spiritual battle.

I turned around to see him and he asked, "Are you not singing Miracles tonight?" I whispered with all the sound I could produce, "I don't think they want me to sing like this!" we chuckled together.

"I believe you are anointed to sing that song, Tim." Rod got very serious with me for a moment, which is uncommon between the two of us. "I am going to go get some oil and a couple of people and I would like to pray over you about this! Would that be ok with you?" What was I going to say to Rod Johnson when he said he wanted to pray over me? He instructed me to stay right there and wait for his return.

In a few minutes, he came into the room with two others and a jug of cooking oil. You read that right. Cooking oil. An entire gallon of cooking oil from the church kitchen no doubt. I nervously glanced at the gallon in his hand.

"I couldn't find any anointing oil. I'm not sure what Pastor Davis has done with it, so, we prayed over this and we are going to use it instead." I was beginning to wonder just how much "anointing" was about to happen!

"I trust you, Rod. If you say you're good with that, then I'm good with that," I whispered.

"Sit down in this chair," He told me flatly as he slid a chair in front of him. He then turned the cooking oil up and let a small amount pour into his hand. He clapped his hands together and placed both hands on my head. I felt the oil on my temples and the other two people put their hands on me as Rod began to pray. I wish I could recall the words he used. I know he told satan where to go and he called on the name of Jesus for a miracle to immediately heal my voice. Other than that, I don't remember anything else. I am sure his prayer over me ended something like, "In the STRONG name of JESUS, AMEN!"

"Now, sing!" He snapped. I just sat there and stared at him. I didn't feel any different and I was pretty sure my voice was still gone.

I started to tell him, "Rod, I want to believe like you.."

"Don't SPEAK! SING!" Rod commanded.

My mind was reeling. I sat there for a second looking bewildered at him. I thought of the words to the song, I opened my mouth and started trying to sing them.

"Many nights we prayed....." I sang. It came out as loud and clear and pure as any night I had sung it before. My eyes widened and filled with tears. Rod just busted out laughing with the others. I couldn't talk, but I could sing.

We rushed out to talk to Karen and inform her. With Rod

beside me I walked up to her. Rod stood there grinning like the Cheshire Cat. I sang for Karen. Her eyes popped open as widely as mine had. She shouted, "Go tell Brooke and go get dressed! Hurry!"

In a moment I stepped into the room where Brooke was practicing my song. She stopped and gave me that look. You know the one, when you interrupt a woman doing something that has suddenly been sprung upon her and she had very little time to prepare for... Rod said, "Sing, Tim." I burst into song. Brooke just stood there looking at me. The look changed to " You have got to be kidding me, right now." "Well, go get dressed!" she said sharply.

I went alone into the room where all the costumes were stored on racks. The lights were out but the windows were open so there was plenty of light butthe room was still dim. I walked across the floor towards the rack that contained my costume. I was dumbfounded. Confusion and giddiness muddled together as I walked. I was full of wonder and gratitude at the same time.

Suddenly, the familiar "still, small voice" that people speak of, quietly, yet firmly, spoke into my heart. "Don't ever doubt me again." It was soft yet crushing.

So many of the moments, when I had questioned His existence, if we were all here just circumstantially, if it all was real, flooded my memory. Played back into my mind's eye in the split of a second, the thoughts, the doubts, the failing bits of time whirled around me, mockingly. They were like demons flying around my head screaming, "You're not a REAL believer! You are full of doubt!" Promptly, their mocking became shrieks of terror as they were vanquished from my presence. I sat down to bear the weight of what He had said. The sobs came in waves as I asked for forgiveness for my lack of faith. My face streamed with tears as I was brought to a place of knowledge. Faith doesn't even describe it. I simply just knew. I knew, in that instant that God is there. He is real. He wants to interact with us. I knew it like I knew the sun was shining. I knew it like I know I am sitting here, typing this to you. My faith was made easy. I still couldn't talk. But, I could sing, and sing I did that night. My voice was completely restored the next day.

I write all of this to help you understand God IS involved and He DOES care. I cannot explain some things that happen. I cannot explain why you are going through what you are going through. The cold, hard, fact is; there are people reading this who will watch their loved one pass away. You will believe He is going to do something miraculous and you will be filled with faith and hope only to watch your child, or mother, or grandfather, or even yourself, lose the battle with some kind of illness. I cannot explain any of that, I am not a prophet or the son of a prophet. I am not a faith healer nor do I claim to have anything special, other than I am a son of a living, loving God. I do not know how to explain why some will receive a miracle and some will not. But I believe in a God who still performs miracles and is more powerful than cancer. I only hope that the testimony of the last few chapters, helps you to have faith in The God of Abraham, Isaac, and Israel, The Father of Christ Jesus who IS the great healer. I for one, will stand up and risk being called a fool, if it means I pray for one hundred people only to see one miraculous healing from that group. I will not be swayed from the belief that God still heals and wants to heal every single sick person and will be glorified through any and all that are healed.

FOURTEEN

SETBACKS AND HURDLES

October 17, 2018 Wednesday morning. It seemed as though I was losing the battle for Heidi and Winston was getting worse. Although I was believing for both of them, praying over them and anointing them both with oil, I was watching Heidi's life and joy deteriorate rapidly. All I could hear was His voice in my head, "..set backs and hurdles…" My heart didn't want to believe it, my head couldn't stop the words of Dr. Rutland from running over and over. "…to me, it sounds like both of your dogs are going to die…." My faith wanted to see them better. My heart wanted at least the words of our friend, Teniece, to be right, "…a set back is something that knocks you off your feet, but a hurdle is designed for you to get over!" Either way, I lay in bed and poured my heart out to the world of Facebook friends again.

Facebook Post October 17, 2018:

"As I lay here, waiting for sleep to find me, I know I am in the hands of God, our graceful Father. I have seen and heard Him move, in the last few weeks, in ways I haven't witnessed in my entire life. Yet, I'm at unrest as Heidi, our German Short Haired Pointer, slowly, unmercifully, fades toward what seems like her untimely death. I thought we might be watching Winston die by now, not Heidi. But, her kidneys are failing and it seems our prayers for her to stay with us for a bit longer are going to be answered with a "No." As a puppy, AdleHeidis Von Ruberta, aka Heidi, immediately became a source of love and laughter for our household. Full of sweet character, inquisitive personality, and psychological nuances never known by me, in any other dog before her, Heidi stole our hearts. My dreams of hunting quail were squashed as she became gun shy suddenly at about 6 months old. But the die were cast and she was firmly rooted into the hearts of the girls in this house, so worker dog or not, Heidi was staying. Among many times of trouble, there was the moment she scared us all to death as she jumped off the waterfalls because she didn't like that we were at the bottom and she wasn't, regardless of the fact that she had ran up the trail to the top. She was our "clearance puppy" that elevated herself to princess status. She required a constant supply of stuffed animals which she could take care of. She needed a chew everyday although she seemed to enjoy taking it and hiding it more than she enjoyed chewing it. She would carry it around like a cigar for hours just to tease Winston. She demanded his attention and loved him with a bond I've never seen between two dogs.

Over the years, she has entertained us with her wonderfully sweet nature. I can only hope we have been for her what she has been for us.

I don't know if dogs go to heaven. I have my doubts, but, if they don't, then heaven will surely be missing a great opportunity to have a wonderful pup there, If they don't, and our only experiences with Heidi are about to be only memories, then I thank The Lord that we had the incredible opportunity and responsibility to be her human guardians for her life. I hope you all have, at least once in your life, the chance to be blessed by an animal's life as we have.

Heidi, thank you for being such a wonderful pet and family member. Thank you for all those "turned head" looks. Thank you for all the lizards you pointed. Thank you for the one bird you pointed for me. Thank you for all the nuisance deer and squirrels you chased from the yard. Thank you for all the wet toys you laid on our laps. Thank you for all the "beetlejuice" back scratches you did in the living room. (Inside term in our house). Thank you, most of all, for being our clearance puppy that won our hearts, ruled our house, and provided us with heart warming memories. We love you."

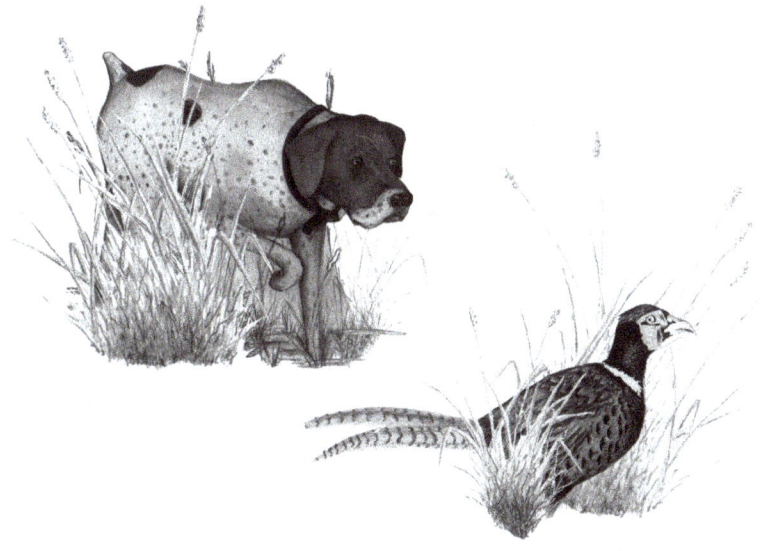

FIFTEEN

WHEN OUR PRAYERS DO NOT SEEM TO WORK

And that was that. The next day Heidi was gone. The cold hard truth was all the praying, the annointing with oil, the hope that she would pull through, the changing of her diet, was to no avail. Sadly, I use the word "hope" instead of "faith" because somewhere deep inside me I had a gut feeling she would die. It was a long, drawn out, downward spiral and although I prayed over her, I never felt as if it was going to change. It still boggles my mind a little. I laid my hands on Winston, watching him get worse and worse, knowing what the vets had told me, knowing that he should be the one who died first. How could I pray over him and be filled with such faith and move five feet away, and pray over Heidi and feel like I was simply uttering meaningless words with powerless religiosity? I can't answer that question. That is the hardest thing about faith and healing. We are not Jesus. There is no story in which we read of Jesus praying over a sick or even a dead person who wasn't healed. There is, however, a story where the disciples try to cast out a demon and could not cast it out. You can find the story in Matthew 17:14, Mark 9:14, and Luke 9:37. I list all three, because to understand the story in full detail, one needs to read all three accounts. I do not want to get too side-tracked here, but there were several aspects of this story that were important to me as I struggled through all of this.

A man comes to Jesus saying he had a son whom he assumed was vexed with a demonic spirit. He said the demon would throw him down in convulsions and had thrown him into the fire as well as into water, trying to kill the child. He had brought the child to Jesus' disciples, yet they had prayed to no avail. Mark records a conversation between the man and Jesus which I found particularly helpful. He says to Jesus, "If you can, please help." Jesus says, "Everything is possible, if you can believe." He replies to Jesus, "I believe! Help my unbelief!" I think that is one of the most real statements in the entire Bible. It described my level of faith perfectly. I believed that God would heal Winston. But I needed a LOT of help with all the parts of me which struggled to believe.

Jesus went on to cast out the demon, and the boy was healed. Later on, the disciples asked why they could not cast it out, and Jesus broke it down for them. First, He said, "Because you have so little faith." He then said, "If you had faith the size of a mustard seed, you could move a mountain." However, He added, "This kind only goes out by prayer and fasting." At first, I thought His answer contradicted itself. As in, "You had too little faith, but, only with prayer and fasting could you have done it." However, if you allow me a little license, I'll add some words in parenthesis to help this make more sense. I understand, I tread on the dangerous ground of presumption. "You didn't have faith enough to cast it out," (but, even if you did have enough faith,) this kind only goes out after you have been fasting and praying." Now, let me rearrange His words to make even more sense. "You had too little faith" *because* "you have not been fasting and praying. with faith the size of a mustard seed," (the size of a mustard seed was a relative dimension they could have understood, basically, one of the smallest seeds imaginable) "you could tell this mountain," (one of the largest, most immovable, ominous things imaginable) "to move and it would do so." (Therefore, if you want that kind of power in your life, you're going to have to fast and pray.) I do not want to chase a theological rabbit here for long. I believe, fasting had something to do with this process. I want to further discuss fasting before I move on.

While praying and fasting for Winston and Heidi, I was discussing the idea of fasting with my friend, Rico. I asked him, "Why," in his opinion, "fasting would or could have made a difference in Winston's situation?" He made this statement. "Fasting creates an atmosphere that shuts down the noise of the world, so we can focus on the Father." I have heard this explained a different way; Think of yourself like an onion. An onion can sit on your counter-top and you can walk by it day after day and you cannot smell it. But, start peeling away the layers and the smell becomes quite strong in the room. Did the onion get stronger? No. The aroma of the onion was locked inside all along. Only when you began to peel away the outside layers, the aroma of the onion was released. Prayer and fasting does this very thing. It separates you from the world, for God. If God's Spirit, that is, The Holy Spirit, is within you, it is as strong as it was the day He came to reside within you. The strength of the Spirit is the same. But when you pray and fast, you shut out your most basic desires and needs. You focus on praying and listening to the Father; thereby, allowing God to peel away the layers of you, the human you, and expose His Spirit living within you. Then His aroma is released in your life. Prayer and fasting doesn't make *you* stronger. It makes *you* weaker so that

His Spirit can operate through you, less obstructed. I am sure the disciples lived holy lives, at least as much, or more than any group of men in history. However, Jesus saw the loose stitch in the fabric of their faith. He knew the depth of their hearts, and He also knew what kind of strength it was going to take for them to face their future. He was encouraging them to live every second, of every day, in communication with the Father. He knew they struggled with mindsets of envy and hope for political conquest and power. He knew those mindsets needed reforming. He wanted them to be able to speak to the mountains they would face, with authority, and see them move. He wants that for us, too. He gave us authority over sickness, disease, and demonic power. Yet, so many of us lack the discipline to be in constant contact with the Father. We then lack the power-filled faith to chase the mountains away. Nor are we willing to fast the things that separate us from God. These things, then, become tools used by the enemy, to point to our weakness and humanity. Satan can bring these up to us and claim we have no right to ask anything of The Creator of the Universe. We must understand this; we are His children. In this alone we have the right to ask of Him. When we spend time fasting and praying it does not make Him stronger. It helps to increase our faith in Him. It helps us to hear Him and feel Him more clearly. Which then increases our faith in Him. If the devil can say anything to us that will keep us from asking, he has already won the battle over faith. Fasting and Praying shuts the noise down from him and reminds us that our Father is with us.

In the midst of this we must still remember, God is sovereign. This is not an "if - then" proposition. If I live this way, then God must perform that way. That is a recipe or formula. I am not describing a spell or incantation, in which we mumble the right words to God and spend so many days fasting, then, when we have reached the pinnacle of our magical chanting, God swoops in with a miracle. Nor, am I setting the stage for healing, as a result of manipulation. God will not be commanded, nor will He be manipulated. We do not have the power within us to direct the creator of the universe to do something that is outside of His will. The flip side of that coin is that sometimes, God does not require a person to do more than simply ask, and He works, on their behalf, a miracle. Why? Because He is like... God. Does that mean that if we pray for healing, for ourselves or for someone else, and it doesn't happen immediately, we should just chalk it up as God's sovereignty and assume He isn't going to heal them? By no means! Jesus gave us an example of praying more than once for healing. Let's take a look at that story.

THE POWER OF PERSISTENCE

In Mark 8, starting in verse 22 we find a group of people bringing a blind guy to Jesus asking for his healing. Jesus takes the man outside the village to work with him privately. Jesus then did something quite odd. It is the only place recorded in the Bible he actually spit on someone. He used his spit to make mud once to heal another blind person. He even spit on his own fingers and touched a man's tongue, (which grosses me out) but in this case, according to Mark, he spat on the man's eyes. Then, he placed his hands on his eyes. Then, Jesus did something that he never did anywhere else, he asked the man about his condition. In Verse 23, He asked him, "Do you see anything?" Forgive my humanity once again, but that question at first, seems odd to me. Jesus, the guy who raised people from the dead from a distance, spits on a man's eyes, rubs it in, and then says, "Are you ok? How's that feeling? Did it work?" Nowhere else did he do anything like this. We don't see him asking the lame man who never walked before, "Hey buddy, do you need help getting home? Those new wheels you have may be a little wobbly at first!" He just did things like forgave their sins, told them to get up and sent them home. Other times he touched them, yet other times he told other people that their loved one was healed. Why then, in this case, did Jesus ask him if he could see anything? To our surprise the guy says, "Well, kind of...I see men like trees." So, Jesus touches him again. Then his eyes were fully restored, and Jesus sent him home. It is not recorded however that Jesus asked him "How about now? Is that better?" I'm reminded of my first eye test. When it was determined I would need glasses, the doctor slid the thing in front of my eyes and would change the lenses, "Is that better or worse? Sharper or darker? Clearer or fuzzier? Is that better or just bolder?" This was the first recorded eye exam! Jesus spits on the guy, "How about now? Sharper or darker?" I am not purposefully making light of anything here, nor is it my intention to be sacrilegious. My point is this; Jesus had a point to make to the disciples. I believe it is possibly the main reason he removed the man from the village. He needed the disciples to be focused on what was going on, and he didn't want distractions. I believe it was a teaching moment for them about the upcoming conversation about their ability to see clearly. I also believe it was a demonstrative example to point out, sometimes we must be persistent in our faith. We have to follow through. We cannot stop halfway. If you are going to see the miracle in its fullness, you must press on even when it doesn't seem like what we thought it should at first. A noteworthy point is that Jesus took the man out of the village as I just explained. I believe he was trying to get the disciple's attention but there is something else we haven't thoroughly looked at here. The scripture says "..some people brought a blind man..." It does not say some people brought their friend as in the case where the guys opened the roof and let their lame friend down into the room. The details are fuzzy around this part. "People" could have meant just some random people seeking the opportunity to see a miracle.

They heard Jesus was in town (he created a buzz like that, I am guessing) and they may have said, "I sure would like to see him perform a real miracle!" "Yeah, me too! You got anybody sick in your family we can take to him?" "No, but you know ole Charlie is always sitting down there by the front gate begging for a quarter. Let's go get him and see what this Jesus can do!" So, when they bring him out to Jesus he throws the proverbial wrench into the plan by saying, "Excuse us for a moment, we need to step outside."

This is my opinion only. He goes out of the village because he knows the heart of the people. It seems clear in the next few passages "the people" were not present during the miracle. He left them in the village. They brought ole Charlie not because they had compassion nor because they believed in Jesus, they just wanted to see a good magic trick. I cannot prove this. I have no real scriptural basis for this idea, but it seems plain to me that Jesus really didn't want those people to see the miracle. I believe people today often ask for things for the wrong reasons.

Jesus sent the man home and told him specifically not to go back into the village. (Which kind of supports my idea that no one but Jesus, the disciples and the blind guy were there) There are a few times that Jesus healed people privately and told them not to go spreading it around but to keep it on the down-low. We could assume he did not want to bring more attention to himself because it could have stirred the religious leaders to kill him before the appointed time. I don't have a problem with that theory at all. However, it is possible that Jesus did not want those "freshly healed" people to expose themselves to the "nay-sayers" too soon. Jesus says satan's number one job is to steal according to John 10:10. It is possible that through the negative influence of others, tearing down what Jesus had done, those people could have had their miracle stolen. Jesus may have been saying don't go blabbing this all over town, right now, because our humanity needs some time of confirmation without the negativity of other's doubts. The people on the outside were only able to see the end result. Later, the next day, when he walked into town, on his own, waving at them they saw what Jesus had done. The lesson, among many, is that we may see miracles happen in stages. We should keep the faith until it is completed.

Jesus also gave us the analogy of the woman, bugging the judge until he gave her what she wanted. In Luke 18:1-8 He tells us God will answer us when we are persistent. In Luke 11:1-5 He again encouraged His disciples to pray with persistence, to have faith that God will answer your prayers. We should continue to pray for healing. Never give up.

Some may think, "Wait a minute, if God knows all things, then He knows what I need. He certainly knows we need a miracle if my loved one is sick. Why should I have to ask even once, let alone again and again? That doesn't sound very loving to me!" The issue of persistence in prayer can be very perplexing. On one hand, God does know our needs before we ever even approach the throne. That is scriptural; Matthew 6:8, "Do not be like them, for your Father knows what you need before you ask him." Why then, should He need for us to ask, furthermore, why should we need to ask and ask and ask again? Prayerful persistence is about the process. He is constantly teaching and shaping and growing us. First, Christianity, in its core, is about faith. If God just made all things better all the time, creating a utopia of sorts for those who called themselves a Christian, God would simply be a universal genie in the bottle, and it would take no faith what-so-ever to be a believer. We would all grow complacent and would take all His blessings for granted, and it would all spin out of control much like what had happened in the days before Noah. We must ask with faith. Yet again, if we muster the faith it takes to ask and that is all it took, one tiny amount of faith, one question, and "poof" the genie appears and the miracle happens, it would take even less faith the next time. Our focus would quickly change to the results of the gift instead of the giver. Every interaction with the Father has one true purpose... To draw us deeper into relationship with Him.

I heard this in a sermon not long ago. In Mark 10:46-52 We read about Blind Bartimaeus. As Jesus approached the area where Bartimaeus sat daily begging for anything he could receive, for he had been blind from birth, he heard that Christ was coming. He began to call out to Jesus and the people around him (full of normal human compassion) told him to shut up and sit down. He called out all the louder until he gained Jesus' attention. Sound familiar? The woman who touched his garment... "Interrupting faith" Yet, I digress. So, Jesus finally calls Bartimaeus out and heals his blindness. If Bart had listened to the well meaning, good people around him, he would have heard satan's lie. "You're not worth His time. It's pointless anyway, your sickness is huge and beyond reach. You've been sick too long. You should just accept your situation and live with it. Shut up. Sit back down and don't bother the important people."

He cried out over and over. God is not Google. We can't simply type in our request or speak to siri and the answer always just pops up. Often, we too easily quit praying about the things we deem as important in our lives.

Look back at the story in Mark 8. After Jesus had spit on his eyes and touched him, he asked if everything was cool. The guy could have run off partially healed thinking "something is better than nothing." Or he could have been embarrassed. "No one else only gets partially healed, it must be me… don't say anything, everyone will know I have a problem." He could have taken what he had received, but he didn't. He answered honestly. "Well, I know you did what you usually do, but it's not quite perfect." He actually said, "I see men walking around like trees." Our response to God (and ourselves) has to be honest. We have to be willing to admit the truth about our conditions. When you are honest you will find that Jesus will put His hands on you again and again. In these situations, our healing, be it physical, emotional, mental, financial, marital, or relational, our healing will come in stages, through a process.[3]

I am aware I seem a long way from the core of the story here, but I have to go on a bit longer about persistence. Could you stay with me for a few more minutes on this subject? Sometimes, our faith has to be stubborn. Sometimes, we have to dig in, believing God for something that may seem ludicrous to everyone else around us. There are moments when we have to stand on what we believe God will do for us. Remember, James tells us a wavering faith is like being driven back and forth by the sea and makes us unstable in all our ways! I know it is difficult to stand in bold, belligerent faith, believing in the face of factual evidence that would otherwise indicate the opposite of what we are believing for. When the world tells you to look at the evidence, instead, look at what Jesus told us and exampled for us about being persistent and stubborn in faith. Luke 18 tells us this parable. Jesus was talking to His disciples and they were discussing faith. Jesus told the story of a woman begging a judge for justice against someone who had apparently wronged her. Jesus was specific in pointing out a couple of times that the judge was not a Godly man and didn't care what people thought of him. That is important because it is such a stark contrast to God our Father who does care for us and is good. He goes on to talk about how the woman continued to show up, day after day, regardless of the fact that the judge continued to ignore her requests. Finally, the judge said to himself, "Clearly, she is not going away, I will give her what she is asking for." Her persistence paid off. Jesus didn't tell us this to say The Father was like the unjust judge. God does not sit and ignore us, and then finally do what we want out of exasperation. Rather, He told us this to describe how we must persist, for whatever reason, until God moves. Go back, with stubborn faith, and ask God, over and over, until you see the evidence of your faith. If you're asking yourself right now, "Why wouldn't God just do it the first time, when we ask in faith, if He is going to do it eventually anyway?" I don't have the answer. But sometimes, He does. Other times, He moves eventually. I can only assume He has His reasons, His lessons He wants us to learn, the stretching of our faith, the building of our character, and ultimately, His sovereign will.

However, I don't think we can read this parable in Luke 18 without viewing it through the lens of Luke 17 and the rest of chapter 18. Although both of the chapters are divided into small sub-stories and teachings that seem to have little connection, when we look at them all at the same time, there is a theme. Attitude. If we are going to expect great things from The Father there are things we must align with. Now, hear me. I am not giving you a list of "10 things you must do to see a miracle in your life." There is no recipe or formula to make God perform miracles for you. When we begin to think that way, we are in danger of putting these things above God and His sovereign will. When we think, "If God is going to do this great thing in my life, I must do (fill in the blank) to ensure he does it. Suddenly, our action becomes greater than God. He then becomes a genie in a bottle for us and is reliant upon our actions for Him to work. It simply does not work like that. However..... and you knew there was a "however" coming right? God DOES require us, very often, to be involved. Obviously, God can do what God wants to do. He wants to do it, and I cannot explain why or when He will act quickly or slowly, or at all, for that matter. But, I believe He will, always, act and I pray and believe as if He will always act immediately and exactly how I am asking. It is the only way I know how to believe.

Having that been said, look back at Luke 17 and 18, Jesus describes attitudes of great faith, gratitude, expectancy graced with humbleness. He suggests persistence bathed in obedience and respect for authority and rules. He urges us to call on him with generosity, mercy, forgiveness, strength and the courage to simply ask. I believe, if there were a formula for seeing God move in miraculous ways, that would be it. But, wouldn't that be the formula for everything Christian? God does not respond because of our formulas, but He often responds to them. He is not a genie where we can simply beckon Him to our every whim. His sovereign will is ultimately greater than our requests, but He is also a good, good father. He hears us and loves us. He cares about things that are important to us. He expects us to do the things on our end that Jesus mapped out for us, with the right heart. And, He knows our genuine intentions and heart when it comes to following these things. I simply can't explain this better.

A PAIR OF STUMBLING BLOCKS

I want to move on with the story here, but I simply must add these two, very real, stumbling blocks we may face. I believe these are both lies from satan, that we may deal with, any time God asks us to pray for someone. The first stumbling block to our faith is: "Who do you think you are?" I believe satan whispers this into our ears when we begin to think that we can pray for someone's healing. "Do you think you're Jesus? Do you think you actually have this kind of cosmic authority?

You must think you are really special! You're a nobody. You are not God! You cannot tell something like cancer to do anything! You don't have enough faith, you don't live right, you aren't… you can't…you will never be….strong enough to do this." It is all the more difficult when you are praying for a loved one. "These people KNOW you!" the devil will say, " They know your past. They know of most of your mess-ups! They will all think you think you are better than they are! In fact, you DO think you are better than they are don't you? You're a wretched sinner, and everyone here knows it and you know it. Forget this, it will never work!"

Then, you pray for your neighbor, and the next day he calls you up and says "Wow, I feel much better! Thank you!" satan loses, God wins and it's because you simply did what you barely had enough faith to do. Then, stumbling block number two raises its ugly head; "You are AWESOME!"satan will whisper to you. "How great your faith must be! Now, all the people around you are going to be asking you to pray for them! You must have a very special gift! God must really be proud of you, maybe, almost as proud of you as you are! You should have a TV show!" Be VERY CAREFUL not to misapply the glory when you pray for someone or something and healing comes. We are simply the rusty tool that God uses for the moment, allowing us to be a part of HIS miraculous work. He is the healer. He is the miracle worker. He has the power. He gets the glory. All of it. Period. If this level of pride creeps in, the motive behind praying for people gets quite fuzzy, in a self-centered need to be lifted up above others! Compassion fades into desire for gratification and the balance is lost. Tread very lightly when your prayers see success, lest we think something of ourselves we are clearly not. Let's move on with the story.

SIXTEEN

GIVE IT UP TO GET IT

In the midst of Winston's sickness I wondered often, "What can I do? What do I need to give up to get God to do what I want? What can I do to show Him how badly I want this?" Believe me I tried a few things. One, in particular, was almost humorous if it weren't so sad.

Remember, the day I was told Winston was supposed to die within weeks my sister challenged me to fast in order to show God I was serious. I felt she was right and immediately began a fast. That fast lasted from midday on Tuesday until midday on Thursday. I drank nothing but water and did not put a single morsel of food in my body. I had eaten breakfast Tuesday morning at 7:00, and did not eat until about 1:30 pm two days later. Weeks later, when Winston seemed to be getting worse, I wondered if I had broken my fast too soon. Remember, after praying for him at the store, I felt as if God had said to me, "You have done all you can do, it's in my hands now."

We left the store and I asked my dad what to do. "Do I just keep on fasting until he stops limping?" He reminded me of what I felt God had just said about having done all *I could do* and we promptly went to eat. I felt like my fast was over. Yet, weeks later, I second-guessed my self. During that initial fast I never felt a single hunger pang. I was never even tempted to eat. I was fasting, that was that and it didn't bother me in the least. In fact, I wondered what the big deal was that I had heard people talk about. It was like I was being protected from what I thought should have been happening to my body, going without any nourishment for a long period of time. Yet, after a few weeks, Winston wasn't getting any better. (Yes, *weeks later*, it's a good thing I didn't think, "keep fasting until he isn't limping.") I began to pray about it, asking God if I had done it all wrong. Suggesting maybe I had broken my fast too soon, maybe I had "wimped out." One morning I was up early again, praying, and these thoughts were running through my mind and I believe God said, "You did what I asked you to do. You fasted for the same amount of time that my son was dead, I think that is sufficient." I stopped in the middle of my prayer time and began to calculate. Jesus died at the 9th hour which is approximately 3- o'clock on Friday afternoon. He rose again at daybreak, approximately 6:00 a.m. on Sunday. Approximately 36 hours had passed from his death to his rising. But in the original Hebrew, because he died on Friday before sundown, Friday was counted as a full day. In their cultural perspective any portion of a day is counted as a day. He lay instate all day Saturday and rose again after the day had begun on Sunday. Once again, any portion of a day is considered a day, therefore "three days later" he rose. I started my fast, technically, around lunch on Tuesday, although it had been around 7:30 am since I had eaten a thing. I ended the fast 48 hours (the third day) from the same perspective the Gospels were written. In my heart, God said, "Your time was sufficient." I pondered the answer, I believe God gave, and was satisfied with what was being revealed to me. Yet, in my efforts to *really prove something* to God, I decided to fast again. Note that I make the distinction between the two incidences. I believed God, through my sister's advice/challenge, told me to fast and pray, the first time. The second time, I am absolutely sure that I simply decided to fast on my own, and in retrospect, I may have been attempting to manipulate God. I started the next day. When I say I was miserably hungry for three days, I fall short of the description as if I was describing the grand canyon as a little ditch with a creek running through it. I even compromised, slightly, by drinking a few protein shakes throughout the three days. I had head aches. I was sick at my stomach. I ached and cramped all over. I had spells of feeling quite "faint". I was light headed and nauseated. I thought I would go insane when my family ate around me. It was just as I imagined going three days without food would be! Clearly, I was fasting without His help or provision, and it was evident He didn't ask me to do this. At some point, in the midst of the three days, I spoke with my friend, Rico, about it all. Rico told me, "If you don't feel like God led you to fast, you're not fasting, you're simply going without food. It won't do you any good anyway." Either way, I don't think I proved anything to God, nor was He manipulated. The only changes I saw in Winston were changes for the worse.

As frustrated as I was, I had to laugh at myself. My poor wife watched me as I struggled through these things. She probably wondered what I might try next. I am sure she walked away at times shaking her head. She always supported me, she never mocked me, she never told me I was crazy. She did her best to encourage me, although I am sure she wanted to shake me violently at times. Long was the list of attempts to shape the atmosphere of our home, to one of healing. I changed his diet. I emptied the house of any alcohol. There was hardly a time there wasn't praise and worship music flowing from some room, especially the room Winston occupied. Our dialog changed in our house for the better, and open, regular prayer became a normality. Not that we didn't pray before this, but not with the regularity in which we prayed then. Do I believe all of those things were a waste? Not at all. All of those things were good changes that needed to happen. All of these things had a purpose in my life that eventually found their balances within reality and spirituality. Let me explain further.

I am not of the religious opinion that any consumption of alcohol in general, is particularly sinful. I am aware there are going to be readers of this from both ends of the spectrum on this point, I am not trying to start a fight here, save your letters. There are Christians who believe a drop of alcohol is a drop too much and it is sinful by the very nature of its existence. Clearly, the over-consumption of alcohol has a very destructive force. We can see it in the marriages, relationships, careers, ministries, and lives which have been destroyed from abuse of alcohol. There is no argument that can sway the blatant facts and obvious dangers of drinking; DUI stats; health problems, child/spouse abuse; all have their connections. However, controlled use of alcohol can even have some health benefits. i.e. A small amount of red wine, regularly, can help your heart. Beer, in controlled amounts, can benefit your urinary tract. Stress can be relieved by the consumption of a small amount of any kind of alcohol. I am not here to discuss the religious legality of consuming alcohol. This is simply part of my story.

I have a particular affection for rum. My personal favorite is spiced rum. I have to be careful with rum however, because, I like it too much. My personal conviction is when I think, "I NEED to have a glass of rum or a beer or wine." I simply will not. I do not want to be *controlled* or dictated by anything other than God. It is also my personal conviction not to drink to get "buzzed" or drunk. Have I ever had too much and ended up there? Yes. However, it is my conviction to stay away from there as much as possible. Yet, I digress.

A popular rum manufacturer released a commemorative bottle of spiced rum called 1671, a number of years ago. Karen heard about it, and knowing my preferences, she bought some for me. I was enamored by its taste. It was, by far, the best I had ever had. A couple of years passed and I wanted to get a bottle of it for my brother for a birthday gift. It had been some time since I had purchased any, so, when I went to get it, they told me it had been discontinued because it was a commemorative run and the company had phased it out. Well, my heart was a little broken but I called around and found some. When I arrived, the guy had 13 bottles of it and to my spouse's surprise and possible slight irritation, I purchased every one of them. What can I say? I really liked it and I had just come to the knowledge there would never be any more available. Luckily, it wasn't terribly expensive. Fast forward a year. I was sitting in church, listening to Travis preach about personal sacrifice and giving everything to The Lord. This was something I have been dealing with since I was young. By nature, I am a little bit of a hoarder (if you couldn't tell, by the first part of this story).

In a moment of self reflection I thought, "Yes, I have given everything to God. If He asked me to sell or give away everything, go to some foreign country to be a missionary, do whatever, it's His and I would gladly go and do whatever He asks of me."

Then came that "still, small voice" people talk about. "Would you get rid of your rum you love so much?"

I was taken aback a little. "That came from no-where" I thought. "Of course. God, you know my heart. I would give it all away if that is what you asked of me." There. It was settled.

I held nothing back from The Father. But somewhere, deep within the recesses of my heart, I truly hoped He never asked me to get rid of it. Months passed and there I was again, sitting in my normal seat, during an altar call, at church, and it came up again.

"I don't believe you would get rid of the rum if I asked you to." I believe God said, and He continued, "and by the way, why would I ask you to give it to someone if that could be a stumbling block to them? Not everyone has control of the drinking issue like you, I wouldn't want you to give it others. That is simply an extension of your hoarding problem anyway. You would be alright, inside your heart, to give it away because it would still serve a purpose for you, in a way. If I asked you to pour it out as a testament of your level of sacrifice to me, would you do that?"

These are the kinds of conversations I have with God sometimes. This question dug at me to my core. He was right. If I gave it away, I could at least know that it was going to be enjoyed by someone I cared about. I had given a few of the bottles to family members anyway. But I didn't know if I could walk in there and open the rest of it and pour it down the drain. The fibers of my inner being were challenged by this thought. Not only would I be destroying the last of my favorite rum, but I would be simply wasting it by pouring it down the drain. I HATE to waste things! (Hence the hoarding issue) I quickly convinced myself I was doing this in my own mind and surely God didn't *really* want me to waste our money and pour out alcohol, with which I truly had no problem! I mean, I rarely had more than one or two glasses, of any alcohol, in a month. Weeks would pass and I wouldn't even think about it. Obviously, I wasn't addicted to alcohol. I felt like this was my own "over-active conscience." Why would He want something like that? The problem was even in the midst of all my arguments, I knew the answer. He would want something like that because He knew, in the depths of my soul, I would have an issue giving it to Him. My problem wasn't with alcohol, my problem was with submission. I held it back from Him. The issue was not my drinking. The issue was my *owning* something I didn't want to give to Him. He could have almost anything from me, and "the hurdle" was the "almost" part of that statement. I told Him that morning I would even pour it out if that was what He wanted. However, it was only lip service, and we both knew it.

Fast forward to a few weeks after Winston was diagnosed with bone cancer. I had begun to pray, I had been to Dalton to get the oil. I had been laying hands on him seeking God's grace and will. Suddenly, one day, I was in the office where the cabinet was that held my rum. I was battling with submitting to the idea that it could be God's will for the dogs to die. I was telling Him, "I don't want them to die, but I will do my best to submit to what you want. I believe you will, in some way, make it work for the good as it says in Romans 8:28. I give it all to you, it is all yours anyway, do with us, in us, through us, what you will." I prayed.

"That's a lie." God said to me.

"A lie???" I was confused and offended.

. "You know what you hold back from me. You know what you are not willing to give to me. You know what you are not willing to sacrifice, if I asked you. You and I know that I can ask you anything….almost."

There it was; The "almost" I had been holding on to and dreading. He wanted me to give Him everything and that meant everything, with no "yes, but not that" attached. With tear filled eyes I gave it to Him. And I meant it. I started to get up and pour it down the drain that moment.

"Wait," I thought I understood Him to say, "Wait for Kaitlyn. I want her to be a part of this, to demonstrate to her the aspect of sacrifice and offering."

"Well, that was a strange command," I thought, but by this time I had begun to get used to "strange commands or requests" by Him. That night, my teenage daughter, Kaitlyn, who loved Heidi as if she were her little baby, helped me pour the last few bottles of 1671 down the drain. We didn't stop there as we emptied the entire house of alcohol that night. I made a commitment not to drink again until I felt as if He released me to do so. If that was never, it would simply have to be never, and I would have to be alright with that. I was. Finally, the thing that held me back from Him was gone.

Unlike my decision to fast the second time, this was not my mind trying to manipulate God. If I had been thinking, "maybe if I do this, He will see how serious I am and heal Winston and Heidi," then, I would feel differently. But, no. This was a spin off issue about which He needed to deal with me. He used the situation to soften me, to make me more pliable to His will. In all of these teaching moments, there was always the notion that it would be the "ta-dah" moment, and the dogs would be healed. Looking back, I simply think He had so many things He needed to teach me, it took this to get me to finally listen.

SEVENTEEN

GOD'S TIMING, BARKING DOGS, AND SHOOTING STARS

Karen and I have always loved watching meteor showers. We have seen some good ones, but the best ones always seemed to be random. In the midst of this learning period, we were getting frustrated. Karen wanted to know more details about the words spoken over us in Puerto Rico. She wanted to know what God has in store for us and our ministry. Was there actually going to be a "ministry?" Sometimes, waiting on God to fill in all the blanks can be mind-wrenching. I am a little more "go with the flow" than she is. She wants a plan and the answers and forward motion. It must drive her insane to be with a guy who always says, "Don't sweat it, it'll work itself out."

I was out of town and she doesn't sleep well when I am out of town. She had been up searching the Internet for ideas for Kaitlyn's wedding. It was very odd, VERY odd, for her to be up past 10. It was nearly 1 a.m. and she had finally decided to try and get some sleep. Lights out and laying down, she lay there in the dark and suddenly Winston jumped up and started barking and growling at the back window which overlooks our back yard. The neighbor's dogs were barking ferociously, as well. We are used to them barking at everything but, this time, they were losing their minds. Because of some dense woods, Winston and the other dogs could not have been seeing the same thing at the same time. I suppose Winston could have been simply riled up from the sound of them, but whatever it was, it had all of them stirred. This behavior from Winston was extremely abnormal. I don't think I have ever seen him get up in the night and bark and growl at anything. She pulled her pistol out of the dresser and laid it on the nightstand and got up to look out the window. "What are you so upset about Wincy?" (her pet name for Winston) She pushed the blinds out of her way and as she peered into the dark. Suddenly, a bright shooting star flashed across the sky from one side of the horizon to the other. She was struck by its beauty.

"Wow, what great timing!" She thought.

Allow me to interject this in the middle of her story. First, all the dogs were doing something they had not done in 10 years. Second, Karen was up at an hour which, I don't think, I ever remember her being up unless we were out for some specific reason. Third, she was awake while I was out of town. This is UN-HEARD of! Fourth, she got up and took her pistol out of the drawer, which took a very specific amount of time. As far as I know, she has never done that before! Fifth, she walked to the window and opened the blinds which is strangely against her nature. In order to grasp the odds against all of this, you also must know the back of our house doesn't have a huge view of the sky. There is a rather small window of trajectory in which it could have been seen, especially for a long track across the sky. There were so many things that had to line up perfectly that were completely out of normal behavior patterns. It is a stretch to think this was a simple coincidence. Not to mention, that meteor has been flying around for an untold numbers of years. Whether you believe it has been floating through space for a few thousand years or millions of years, it "just-so-happened" to break into our night sky at the perfect location for her to observe its flight. It "just so happened" to fall into our atmosphere at the perfect time for all of these things to have caused her to be standing at the back window, peering into the night sky. Coincidence? Maybe. But, I don't think so. Yet, I digress once again.

"Wow, what great timing." She thought. And right there, standing at the back window, peering into the dark, night sky, at 1:00 a.m. Karen heard His still small voice.

"In my time." He said.

She understood Him to be saying, "We will do all things in my time. I've got you." The dogs settled down immediately. She calmly walked back to the dresser, put away her pistol, climbed in bed, and slept like a baby.

It was yet another class completed in this crash course of faith, listening, trusting, and acting accordingly. A master's level class in paying attention and self-examination. Far be it from me to think we have earned some degree in any of this, but we have certainly learned from it!

EIGHTEEN

SURREALITY OF DECEMBER

Humanity sucks sometimes. In spite of all the faith I could muster, so often I would watch Winston struggle to get up, hop over to the door or his water bowl, and it would break my heart. I could almost physically feel it. The disappointment and crushing thoughts that would start out as a sinister chuckle in the back of my head. "He's never gonna be ok. He has cancer, and you know he is going to doing something to cause that leg to shatter, and you are going to look like the biggest fool of them all with all your 'faith-filled' words and all your 'Godly' predictions!" My spirit would rise up to squelch all this banter. However, some days, it was too loud. It is the forefront of the battle between spirituality and humanity. There were days that I had prayed with all the faith and strength I could muster and then, on the verge of giving up, out of the blue, I would get a call from John Jennings. Clearly, it could have been coincidence that John would call me when I was at my lowest. I choose to believe it was God, providing for me the comfort and encouragement I needed.

He would, invariably, ask how Winston was doing, and I would try and answer with faith saying, "He is still limping, but I am still believing that God is going to do something."

John would say things like, "Your eyes are seeing him limp, but what you see is not what you have to believe. Our eyes are full of lies. We walk by faith and not by sight! You are a son of the Living God! What He says is what goes, not what that lying disease is trying to say. That disease has no business in your house or in your family! Tell it to leave. Tell it there is no room for its existence where the Children of God reside! We are going to see the miraculous Hand of God in this!"

I wanted so badly, to believe like that and I stood right on the crisp edge of that kind of faith, yet my humanity screamed, "That kind of thing only happens to guys like John! Not guys like you who have normal, earthly, sinful struggles in your life!" This is yet another tactic, from satan, of killing your faith.

Surreal: Webster defines this word as: *marked by the intense irrational reality of a dream: unbelievable, fantastic.*

December 1, 2018, I was in the front yard, doing some work on the bushes. Winston was outside with me, as is normal for the two of us. Even though he limped everywhere he went, if I was outside, he wanted to be outside. I was near the front right corner of the house, and he came around from the driveway and crossed the front yard behind me. In the corner of my eye I caught him, and I stopped trimming the bushes and stared. I remember it as if it were in slow motion. He just went about his business as usual, trotting across the yard towards the other side of the house... Without limping. I sat the trimmers down on the sidewalk and began to follow him, trying not to be noticed, so I could watch without stirring him up. I followed as closely as I could, staring at his right leg, as he went. Full pressure, walking with a normal gait, no limping. Chills ran up my spine, from excitement. My heart pounded and my breath came to me as if I had run down the street. I continued to follow and watch. I am not sure for how long. Tears welled up in my eyes and my face was frozen into an uncontrollable smile. It was truly surreal. I am not sure why we believe for something great, we claim it, we pray for it, we tell ourselves and everyone, "Well, this is what I think is going to happen..." and everyone thinks you are crazy for thinking and believing for the thing that seems against all odds. You are willing to be thought of as crazy because you believe it, so strongly, and then, when it actually comes to fruition, you stand there, mouth agape and think to yourself, "That is incredible, I can't believe it!" I walked around behind him, and I could barely believe what I was seeing. I waited for the hammer to fall. I waited for him to turn back and lift his leg up and hop back toward the door, as if there was some cosmic joke going on and the whole universe was going to laugh and say, "Just kidding!"

I wish I could say, having seen the result of strength and steadfast persistence, my faith was bolstered; I wish I could say I stuck my chest out, with confidence in my Heavenly Father, ready to tell the world, "I told you God was going to heal him!" But that wasn't me. That hasn't been me for a year. I *was* filled with faith that God was going to heal him. I *did* believe it with all that I could muster. I *had* seen God's hand moving unnervingly through my life, in the recent months. I had *no reason* to doubt God. I *was* proud that God had come through in this incredible moment. I was all of those things, and yet I couldn't believe it was happening and especially happening to me! Somewhere, deep inside, I think I was convinced that God *could* heal Winston, and God *wanted* to heal Winston, but there is an inherent flaw in my existence that would screw that up, somehow, because ultimately I didn't deserve that kind of favor from The Father. So, when Winston was walking with no limp, I held my breath for something to go wrong. Remember the idea of prayerful persistence? I prayed every single day, many times more than once, over Winston, for 105 days. I asked God for a miracle while watching Winston get worse and watching Heidi die. I could not make sense of it all, yet I was seeing the results of the process before my eyes. I don't tell you this to pat myself on the back. Hopefully, you know that much about me, by now. I tell you that as a testament of the process of persistence.

He showed absolutely no signs of any pain yet, I kept watching him for days, waiting for the limp to come back. He just kept walking normally. On Dec 11, I video taped him jumping and running. He put so much pressure on his leg I thought, for sure, it would snap. I was so nervous while watching him bounce around, I had to make him stop. He continued to play and run every chance he had. He must have been filled with joy to finally be able to romp around that way again. Against Karen's advice, four days later, we went duck hunting. He retrieved four ducks that morning, one of which was at least 60 yards away in the water. He swam like a champ, as if nothing had ever happened. I must admit, I held my breath every time he entered the water. His greatest challenge would come 5 days later.

Because I make duck calls, I have a connection with an organization named Hunting for The Cure (HFTC). HFTC is made up of a great group of people who take kids with cancer, and their families, on hunting and fishing trips of a life time. I am honored, occasionally, to guide these families on the duck hunts.

On December 15, I received a phone call from Keith, the founder of HFTC, about guiding a boy who was battling brain cancer. It occurred to me, I had not spoken with Keith about Winston's battle with cancer, and he was oblivious to the previous months of our lives. I was hesitant, simply because these hunts can be quite taxing for a dog in the best of health. (When Winston was about a year old, I guided for HFTC, in the same location, and he retrieved well over 30 ducks that day.) I informed Keith of all that had happened and told him we would be there but, I would have to stop Winston from retrieving if he showed signs of pain. He agreed.

I awoke on Dec 19th, the morning of the hunt, with a fever of over 100 and what seemed to be the onset of the flu. I truly did not want to hunt. I called Keith, concerned that I may introduce some kind of contagious virus to the young man. His parents were quick to say, "The level of antibiotics he was on was so high, there was nothing I could bring that he wouldn't fight off easily." With that, I decided to go. I prayed about my own health and dressed for the cold temperatures. I knew it was going to be a lot of work. I wondered if we would be up to the challenge and I planned on trying to hold Winston back a little. That turned out to be a bit of a joke. He went full steam, wide open. I held my breath most of the day. He retrieved 19 ducks and that afternoon I could barely tell he was tired. The young man and his entire family were thrilled about Winston's story of miraculously overcoming bone cancer. It was such a blessing to be able to share it with them and have them there to watch him perform as well as he ever had. I cringed each time he took off or jumped into the lake. My heart skipped a beat to see him sprint down a hill after a wounded duck. I wanted to be completely confident he was fully healed. However, my humanity kept thinking, "This can't be right. Something is going to go wrong." Yet, Winston worked flawlessly. When we got home I thought for sure he would fall out from exhaustion. He was just normal Winston, happy and playful and full of life.

I watched him, with scrutiny, for any signs of pain, for days. He showed none. As far as I could tell, he was healed. God's word to me, had been fulfilled. I was skeptical, but overjoyed.

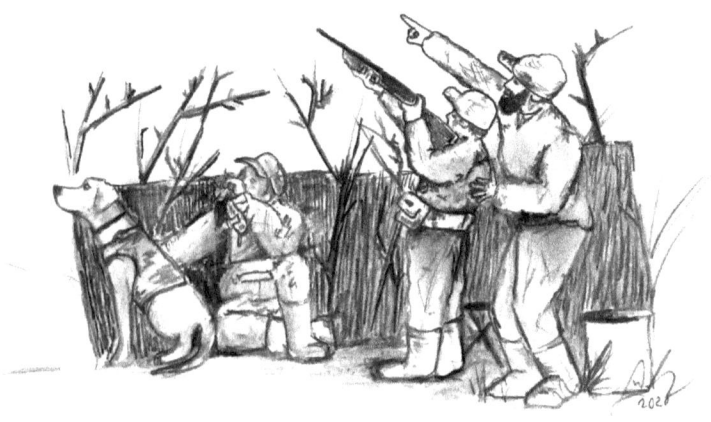

Tim and Winston guiding for Hunting for The Cure

Even after all of this, my spirit battled my mind and I struggled with fear that he would relapse. I mentioned, before, how satan would remind me of my sin, of how I didn't deserve the kind of miracle my friend, John, was talking about. I would hear satan say, "You're not the same kind of guy as John!" I would hear. "John lives every minute for the Lord, you struggle with normal issues and sins. You, Tim, should not expect to see that kind of miracle in your life!"

The voice of truth says something different. The truth is; I AM a child of God and if you have Christ in you, then, so are you. The truth says, "God's grace IS sufficient to cover our sins and wash them away." If our sins are forgiven and "cast as far as the east is from the west," as the scripture tells us, then, my sinful past should have no impact on the outcome of a possible miracle. Yet, this is another thing satan will use (and we don't help ourselves through self condemnation) to create doubt in our minds . He says, "Okay, so you have faith, and okay, you believe God is actually concerned about your tiny little life, but do you actually believe He can do anything in your pitiful existence? Do you think He can work through all that sin in your life? Do you think He will simply ignore how bad you really are? He is holy, you know… and you are… like… *really, not* holy. You do not deserve His grace, His mercy, His blessing and especially a special favor like a miracle!" These things separate us from His miraculous hand because their "noise" can be louder than the voice of Truth and Faith, which resides in us. The Truth says this: 1 John 1:8-9 tells us, "If we claim to be without sin, we deceive ourselves and the truth is not in us. If we confess our sins, he is faithful and just and will forgive us our sins and purify us from all unrighteousness." This is a "If this, then that" statement of promise. If we confess, then He will forgive. Romans 1:17 says, "In Christ, our sins have been forgiven and there is no condemnation." That means, no condemnation from satan, or from your local church, or from your own mind! This doesn't mean we can simply go about living any kind of life we want and throw out "I am not condemned, according to Romans!" We cannot live willy-nilly and expect God to be our "genie in the bottle" when we need healing or blessing or whatever. However, satan's condemnation should fall on deaf ears if we have confessed our sins and asked to be forgiven. He can point to our behavior all he wants, however, under grace, we are forgiven. In addition to grace, when we regularly, through spiritual discipline, fast and pray, the voices of condemnation are silenced. The miraculous, then, has been "set up" through His Grace and by honoring God in our everyday lives.

Then, when my mind, or the demons around me, began to scream, "You don't deserve this!" My spirit can stand up and say, "Tell that to the Father who forgives me and says I do. According to 1 John, what He does with my humanity and sin is His business, not yours! What He chooses to do in my body or in the body of someone I am praying for, is His business, as well, and frankly, I don't remember asking for your opinion!"

For those of you who are like me, who do not do well memorizing scripture and bringing it back up at the moment you are faced with these situations, I have included a list of these scriptures in the back. When our minds or satan throw this lie into the mix, this is the scripture you can answer him with. Take a photo of the page. Tear it out and put it in your wallet or purse. Do *something* so you can reference it, when you need it. You may not have a John Jennings who calls you, out of the blue, to tell you what you need to hear. God did that for me, so I can do this for you. Be strong, He is working. You know how I know? If He was not, you would not have this book in your hands. It is by God's grace and miraculous hand and direction that you have come to read these words. This is not by happenstance. This is Him, moving in your life for YOU. Be encouraged by that.

I would be remiss, at this moment, if I did not say this; If you have never believed on Jesus, as your personal Saviour, the Son of God, the lamb slain for the sins of the world, yours, mine, and all who came before us and all who will come after us; if you have never believed on Him for the salvation of your soul, now is a perfect time to do just that. This book was not written as an attempt to convert people. However, I am writing of things that involve a relationship with the one whom I believe to be the Messiah. I believe Jesus died for my sins and rose again to conquer death, and He ascended to heaven and will return again. I believe I have experienced that Grace in my life. I know that He said He is the only way to The Father, and I have experienced the power and peace of His Spirit residing in me and through my life. People can dismiss all of the words of the Bible and can dismiss the concepts of Christianity and call it "religion." People can deny the evidence set before them and say that science is the only logical answer. They cannot deny one thing: My personal experiences, in my own life. They cannot say, "This or that never happened." They cannot say, "You never heard God's voice in your heart." They cannot say, "You have never seen His hand move." I have experienced God in my life, in a very real and tangible way many times. I know God is real, and I believe He sent His Son to die for me, and He gives me strength and grace to live. I believe Jesus was raised from the dead, to conquer death and sickness, and I believe He is in heaven, awaiting my arrival. If you have never accepted Jesus as your personal Saviour, there is nothing stopping you from doing that right now, before you read another word, before you go another moment, facing whatever it is you may be facing. He is calling you. He said, "Behold, I stand at the door and knock, and if anyone will let me in, I will come in and dine with him and he with me." Revelation 3:20 Let Him in. You can pray these words now; "Father, I believe, help my unbelief! Father, I accept your Son as my Saviour. Forgive my sins, wash me clean and allow me to live, as your child, from this moment on. I believe on Jesus from today forward. Amen." If you just prayed that prayer, welcome to my family. Welcome to the family of God, through Christ. Call someone, and tell them. I don't care who, you can call the nearest church and simply tell them what you just did, or, you can email me and tell me. Confess your salvation to someone, soon.

NINETEEN

MY ISHMAEL

I thought of ending the book with the climactic day of Winton's healing and walking. I cannot. Over the last year, as I have written this, things have taken place connected to "The Story" which I feel, for whatever reason, I am supposed to include. It may be anti-climactic which is not the best idea for your first book! But, this is not like a *normal first book!* With that said, I continue, cautiously, to pour the rest of "The Story" out on you.

Most people know the story of Abraham. Not everyone knows the entire story of Abraham, Sarah, Hagar, Issac and Ishmael. At the time I am writing about, Abraham was still being referred to as Abram and Sarah was actually Sarai, but so we don't get confused, we will keep the names we all know so well. You can read the entire story in Genesis 16-17 but I will lay it out here simply. God had made a promise to Abraham, for years, that he would be the father of a great nation. He promised a son, through his wife Sarah. The problem was Sarah was already in her eighties. Abraham was having a hard time believing his wife was able to bear a child. After all, it had been years since God had made this promise to Abraham, and no kids had been conceived. Sarah decided they should take matters into their own hands. She did the unthinkable. She convinced Abraham to take her maid servant, Hagar, to bed, so Hagar could bear him a son. Abraham gave in, (reluctantly I am sure) and took Hagar to bed with him. However, once Hagar knew she was pregnant, she began to hate Sarah. We are left to assume there was some jealous dynamic going on. No real surprises there! Sarah then blames the entire fiasco on Abraham. Wisely, Abraham tells Sarah, "She's your servant, do what you want with her." So, Sarah begins to reciprocate the hateful behavior. It's not like we couldn't see that coming, right? Hagar decides to bail, and she runs away. She is met by an angel on the road and he tells her she should go back home to Sarah and that her child would be blessed. She did and she bore a son and they named him Ishmael. He was the physical evidence of Abraham's impatience and wavering faith, in God, to do what He said He would do. I am usually hesitant to add anything to scripture, in an attempt to personalize a story, recorded in the Bible. However, in thinking through this, I tried to empathize. I imagine, Abraham justified this in his own mind. He probably thought, "Sarah and I will raise this child as our own. He will be the heir that God was talking about. Sarah is too old to have a child. I am sure God is not going to change that now!" Who knows? Abraham may have even been hearing the lies of satan, "God tried to give her a child many times, but you screwed it up! It's your fault! It was your sin that has caused this. Anyway, that promise was so long ago, if He was going to give her a child, it would have happened long, long ago." Or, satan could have used the one he uses all the time, "You may have mis-heard God!" That lie, the "don't you think, maybe, just maybe, you missed God on this one?" has more depth and power in it than just about any other lie satan can tell us. There are several tactics he uses when making us question whether or not we *really* heard from God. Those questions begin to rise softly, "Are you sure you heard from God? How sure are you that you got it EXACTLY the way you remember it? Is it *possible* that you confused it? Do you know what they are going to think about you if you miss this? You're going to look like the biggest fool!" We can be confident in our salvation. We can know that we know, He has the power to do what He wants, but it is easy to start second guessing ourselves when it comes to "hearing God's voice."

Once again, I am on the dangerous ground of supposition, because Abraham may have literally heard the audible voice of God. There are no indications as to whether God was speaking to him in that "still small voice" through his spirit or if God spoke audibly. Imagine poor old Sarah, barren of children and aging, watching Abraham with young Hagar and *their son* running around the house. What a recipe for disaster. In the next chapter, the story fast forwards 13 years and God tells Abraham again that Sarah will have a child. 13 years had gone by. (Plus all the years before this time they have been waiting.) Sometimes, God's timing makes no sense to us. Sometimes, we have to watch others have what we think we are supposed to have. Sometimes, it feels like what we thought was going to happen, will never happen. Hang on to the faith that God does not lie. Sarah did become pregnant and bore them a son, Isaac. Through Isaac, Abraham did become the father of the Nation of Israel. Also, through Ishmael, he became the father of another great group of people. Those people make up the nations in the middle east, aside from Israel. However, Ishmael's very existence was troublesome and painful for Abraham. From this story, we are supposed to learn these two important lessons; "Don't take things into your own hands and God will come through on His promises."

Did I learn that lesson? A little too late. Right before Winston started walking again, Karen sent me a picture of a cute little black lab puppy. A friend of a friend had a litter of pups and this was the last one. They were willing to cut us a deal, if we wanted it. I knew that the next duck season was a long time away but, I knew I would need a Lab for hunting. I wasn't sure Winston would be up for that, even if he were still alive. I WANTED to have faith that he would be fine, but I was hearing all those lies from satan. I told Karen I was interested in seeing the puppy which she responded to by telling me I didn't need a puppy. She had just sent the picture to me because the pup was so cute and that she knew she had probably made a mistake by sending it. I called the people anyway. Then, December 1 happened, and Winston walked by me without limping. By this time, I had convinced myself that I wanted that pup because "if and when Winston was better, I wanted a pup for breeding purposes. But, my entire family really knew what was going on. I was quietly giving in to the doubt. Even after he walked by me, I set the appointment to go see the puppy. Karen, regrettably, went with me, hoping she could talk me out of it, I am sure. I had preempted her strike by carrying reinforcements. I invited the girls to go with us to see the pup. That was all it really took. We all knew we would not be coming home without the pup. We didn't. Despite all I knew, and all I believed, I wanted to make sure I would have a lab for the next duck season. What was it I said about Ishmael? He was the physical evidence of Abraham's impatience and wavering faith, in God, to do what He said He would do. Enter Sadie.

A couple of weeks went by, and we were at church one Sunday when one of my hunting buddies referred to her as "my Ishmael" and immediately I knew I was busted. He was right. I had taken things into my own hands, despite God's promises I believed I had heard. I had fallen prey to the lie, "If He were going to heal him, He already would have... and what you're seeing, with Winston walking and all... what if it is only temporary? Then what are you going to do?" Either way, I had an Ishmael on my hands, and she was a "holy terror." Let the voice of experience reinforce what you already know. If you believe He told you something, hang on to it. Don't take matters into your own hands. He will come through. He is a good, good Father, and He will finish what He starts. Even when we blow it! At the end of the book, there are a couple of links to youtube videos from our ordeal. The black lab in these videos is Sadie. My Ishmael.

The Winston and friends video:

153

TWENTY

WRITE THE STORY

The right time, the right place, and a rare moment in which Karen and I were together. We were eating in a new establishment in Loganville. I had been watching the construction of the store and wanted to get by and meet the owners. A day or two before, I had dropped by, met the owner (Leslie) for a short period and planned to bring Karen. It was January 25th and Karen and I were already enjoying our meal. I noticed an older gentleman in the official restaurant attire and he was brightly talking to some young ladies who were sitting near the front. He made eye contact with me and moments later, he walked over to our table. He was pleasant as he asked if he get us anything or discard anything for us. I inquired of him, about his job and he explained that he was there to greet people and bless them anyway he could. He introduced himself as Dewitt.

"What a great thing to do!" I commented. "That's a good

idea from the owners. They seem to be such good people." I observed. In a brief moment the conversation turned spiritual, referencing the faith of Leslie and her husband, the owners. How he felt he was there as an ambassador of Christ, to simply love on people. We both clearly recognized each other as Christian brothers, and made more small talk about that. Then, as *normal* conversations would end and the greeter would say, "Well, let me know if I can do anything for you, have a nice day," Dewitt turned back to speak to us.

"I need to tell you," Dewitt said, "The aroma of The Lord is all over the two of you."

I thought, "What a peculiar thing to say." I had never had anyone say anything quite like that to me. For that matter, I have never heard it said about anyone. The "aroma of the Lord," I thought. Karen and I glanced at one another, inquisitively, and then looked back at him. He continued, "You know, the next two years are going to be banner years, financially. God's going to pour Himself out like never before."

Back in the 90's there was a huge media buzz in the Christian World. I'm not a history scholar, so I won't pretend to know a great deal about this. However, in the Jewish calendar, there is a year that comes about called the "Year of Jubilee." It usually marked a great financial year for the Jewish people, when debts were forgiven and the people were bountifully blessed. According to the historical dates, the Year of Jubilee was falling in the 90's, and the Christian church was claiming those promises for themselves, expecting to be blessed greatly during the year. Well, if I was blessed more than usual, I missed it. Maybe there was somewhere, some group of people who were financially set apart that year, but I was not among them. I thought Dewitt may have been among those believers and was referring to something of that nature. I was so convinced of this, my response to him was, "Ohh, I didn't know it was the Year of

Jubilee again."

"No," he retorted, "I'm not talking about all that stuff, I mean for you, the two of you. God is about to bless you mightily, and it's going to start this year."

Again, Karen and I looked at each other strangely. Having heard the preacher in Puerto Rico say "he saw millions of dollars flowing through my hands" and saw Karen "supplying thousands of shoes for children" we were astonished to hear this guy saying this, and frankly, I was becoming a little "weird-ed out." We grinned at each other knowing what the other was thinking. Then looked back at Dewitt. He just stood there, hovering above us with a wide smile on his face. My mouth kind of dropped open because I wanted to speak but was a little dumb-founded. Karen just snickered and we kept looking at him and then back at each other. Finally I was able to formulate some words.

"Uhh, Dewitt was it?"

"Yes". he said.

"You have no idea how significant the words are that you just spoke. We really need to get together and.."

"Habakkuk 2:2." He cut me off mid-sentence.

"Huh?" I questioned.

"Habakkuk 2:2." He repeated. "God says for me to tell you, Habakkuk 2:2."

I chuckled. Slightly embarrassed, I was going to have to admit that I had no idea what that scripture was. I knew there *was* a "Habakkuk" in the Bible but I wasn't sure I had ever read a single word from the book. "What's Habakkuk t..."

"Write the story!" He cut me off again. "Write the vision, clearly. That's what God says for me to tell you."

Now, the partially agape orifice in the front of my face was hanging wide open. All joking aside, my mind had just been blown.

"Write the story." I repeated in my mind. "Of course!" I thought, "I SHOULD write this story!"

Honestly, I cannot recollect anything after that, my mind was reeling so fast about how I needed to get home and start writing this book. I remember telling him we needed to get together so I could explain it all to him. I am sure, Karen was thinking, "That's what Tim needs to do, start another project, especially something as involved as writing a book!" However, as always, she supported me, and somehow it all seemed perfect. I went home and looked it up.

Habakkuk 2:2 Then the LORD *replied:*

2. "Write down the revelations and make it plain on tablets so that a herald may run with it. 3. For the revelation awaits an appointed time; it speaks of the end and will not prove false. Though it linger, wait for it; it will certainly come and will not delay.

After I read the scripture, I started writing. Think about this; You are now reading a book written because a stranger walked up to me, while I was eating lunch and told me, "God said 'Habakkuk 2:2'." Does that feel as strange to you as it does to me?

TWENTY ONE

JUST THE NORMAL KIND OF MIRACULOUS

I need to reiterate something here. I do not write any of this as a testament to myself. I do not tell anyone any of this in order to inflate my ego. I am nothing special except a Christian, saved by Grace. I am nothing great, in any way, other than what Christ makes me to be, a child of The Father, God. I have no room to be egotistical because I cannot claim to have anything to do with the success or failure of prayer. I write this entire book for three reasons. First, because I feel, one hundred percent sure, God directed me to do so. Second, to glorify Him and His miraculous works of grace which I do not deserve and third, to bolster your faith so that you can believe, or start believing, or start trying to believe, in something greater than yourself and science. By the way, any of those stages of belief, or unbelief, are just fine with God. He meets us where we are. God is big enough to handle your wavering belief. I write this to encourage whatever faith you may have.

Here is where we hit the fast forward button and zoom through time. Over the last year, I have had the opportunity to share this story with a number of groups. I have shared with hundreds of individuals. Karen and I have been inundated with strangers, who have come into our lives for brief moments, who were sick, or had a family member sick, with whom we could pray. Often, as I am leaving my home, I feel prompted to go to my cabinet, in my office, and get a bottle of oil. Rarely does that happen that I do not run into someone, that day, who needs to hear the story about Winston's healing, and I give them the bottle of oil that I picked up for them that morning. Just to be clear, I don't walk out everyday and grab a bottle of oil, just in case, then go through the day searching for that person who is sick. I would guess it happens once every couple of weeks, I just feel prompted to bring it with me. I put the oil in my pocket and usually I forget about it, until I am confronted by the person who has a need. It is in that moment, I remember I have the oil, and I give it away. It has become a normal part of my life.

In October of 2018 my dad started feeling poorly. He was losing his energy and having pains that were not normal at all. After a battery of tests and a number of doctor visits, they determined he needed a valve replacement in his heart. His unhealthy condition, however, had rendered him incapable of going through the more routine type of surgery of open heart valve replacement. It was suggested that he be put into a program where they would perform the surgery on his heart through his femoral artery. He would have to enter into a study group to be analyzed for a decade after the surgery because there had only been about 100,000 of these operations performed to date. Insurance had to be approved and finally in January, 2019, he was scheduled for the operation. He was not feeling well at all the morning of the surgery. We were there with mom when the doctors came into the waiting room. They informed us the surgery went fine and the valve was in place and functioning well. However, as they were removing the instruments they perforated something and he was bleeding badly into the pericardium. They had installed a drain with a pump to remove the fluid build up but that was temporary. For the moment, they were going to watch how he progressed, but they suggested they may have to go in and repair the perforation. The problem with that was, he was not healthy enough in the first place to do open heart surgery, and this was radical, emergency open heart surgery, and he was in much worse shape than before the original surgery. They were medicating him to help him sleep, and we should know something in the next 12 to 24 hours. The next day came and mom called. She was quite worried. It was about 11:30, and I was meeting Karen for lunch when she called me. They had come to the conclusion that dad had not one, but likely two perforations. He was not doing well, and the pump was still pulling blood from within the pericardium at an alarming rate. They were trying to got him scheduled for a CT scan but did not know when that would happen. Mom asked if Karen and I would come down to the hospital. We left without hesitation. That morning had been one of those times I felt like I was supposed to have oil with me, but I had no idea I would be seeing my dad. Honestly, I thought he would be fine by noon and probably be released from the hospital. Either way, I had a bottle of oil in my pocket. Karen saw that I had been unnerved by Mom's phone call and suggested she drive for us. I agreed and began to pray in the passenger seat. I believe I heard from God on the way, as we drove in silence.

I believe He told me this, "Go into the room and ask everyone to leave with the exception of Karen. Put the oil on your hand and rub in on your dad's chest. I will tell you how to pray when you start praying."

As I am writing this, something has just occurred to me.

Remember the Sunday morning I referred to earlier, when God told me to go to the stage and say something without revealing to me what He wanted me to say? Remember how I resisted and He continued to push me and worked through Travis and Sylvia to get me to go? I have wondered what the point behind all of that was for me personally. I believe I have just discovered the practical reason He put me through that. He needed to set a precedence in my life, for when He would say, "Go do this, I will fill in the blanks later," then, I would have the faith to step out and do what He said do, despite not having all the details. He needed me to know, "In the moment, He will do what He says He will do." In an effort to be transparent, let me state; I am glad this occurred to me right here, right now, as I write. It tells me He is not finished giving me what we all need to hear and it further demonstrates how He connects it all from the beginning! Clearly, He is still teaching me that if He is going to ask me to go out on a limb, He will already be sitting out there on the limb, waiting on me to arrive, and He will not fail me.

I walked into the room as the male nurse was leaving. Mom was about to leave as well and my siblings had already come and gone to the waiting room. Dad was reclining in a chair and he looked terrible, to be honest. He was gray. His lips were colorless. His eyes were weak and hollow and his voice small and shaky. I never asked Dad, but I am convinced, he was sure that he was dying.

As soon as he realized we were alone in the room he spoke. "Tim, promise me you'll take care of your mother." Those are not the words you want to hear from your dad....ever.

I said, "I do, but you're not gonna need me to take care of her, you're going home to take care of her yourself."

I tried to sound faith-filled, but I was scared to death. I don't think you say those kind of things unless you're convinced that something very bad is going to happen. At best, he believed it certainly could happen. I looked over all the equipment in the room. The little pump which was drawing the blood from his pericardium had a gauge on the front. I am not sure of the units of measure however, I assume it would be "CC". There were little black marker lines drawn on the front to help the nurses track how much blood was being pumped from him. The previous shift nurse had made the mark at around 83. The nurse that had just walked out of the room had marked it at 96. I walked over and told Dad what I believe God had told me and he agreed. I helped him unbutton his shirt, poured some oil into my palm and rubbed it all over the center of his chest. Karen was there with me and placed her hands on him and prayed while I prayed.

I began the prayer, waiting for the words that God had promised He would give me. "Father, you know our hearts…" the words began to flow and I prayed for "any perforations to be closed." I prayed that God would "be magnified and glorified through dad's miraculous healing." I prayed that "at the time of the CT scan they would not be able to find any perforations and that the bleeding would stop immediately." I spoke to his body and told it to "come in line with the scriptures," and I prayed with "the power of the Spirit who raised Christ Jesus from the dead."

That was it, that was all I had, it was all I heard, and I believed it was enough. He was very tired so we decided to let him sleep. Karen and I met with the family in the waiting room. The afternoon dragged on and we caught up with family members as you usually do in situations like that. A couple of times through the afternoon, we spoke to doctors concerning the possibility of them doing the CT scan. Apparently, they were backed up terribly and kept putting him off. He continued to sleep all afternoon. So we let him sleep. Finally at 5:30 they came in and said it was going to be late that night before they got him into the CT scan room. We decided to say our goodbyes and wait for mom to let us know how it went. Karen and I went in to give him a kiss and before I left the room I checked his pump... after 4 hours it hadn't moved one mark. I didn't say anything to him or anyone else about that, I just wanted to observe. On our way out we had to pass the nurses station. I grabbed his male nurse and ask him about the fact that the pump was showing no movement.

His eyes widened and he said, "Well, that's a good thing!"

We went home, and I tried to rest. I was scared for my dad, but I had an odd peace that he really was going to be okay. We were up early, as usual, the next morning. And I waited patiently for my mom to call. At 7:30 that call came in.

She sounded quite chipper and she said, "Well, the CT scan was done at 9:30 last night. They came in this morning to read the findings. They are removing his drain because they couldn't find any perforations during the CT scan! And they plan to send him home at noon today!"

Then he spoke up in the background. He sounded like a different man. In fact, he sounded just like my normal dad. Eighteen hours prior, he sounded like he was at death's door. Now, he sounded as if he could go chop wood. A lot of people would explain this away as coincidence, or the body healing itself, or whatever. I know, and so does my dad, as well as my wife and Mom, God performed a miracle on Dad's body that night. I was just an instrument, a tool. God doesn't need us in order for Him to do miraculous things, but I believe He allows us to be a part of it, to build our own personal faith, so we can share those experiences with others and help build their faith. I do not pretend to understand all the "in's and out's" of why God uses people, or why He calls men and women who are riddled with problems, sin, and all types of afflictions, to do anything. He is God. He is the creator. He doesn't *need* us.

Yet, He communes with us. He asks us to do things, to believe certain ways, to act on His behalf, knowing all the while in our humanity we are very likely to mess it up. Still, He calls us to be a part of something great He wants to do. It boggles my mind sometimes. This rusty old shed tool was brought out of the drawer to be used for something I never thought I was qualified to do. I suppose He qualified me and that's enough.

TWENTY TWO

THE PLAN COMING TOGETHER

The morning of August 25th, 2019 I had what we have come to refer to as a "senior moment." I thought it marked the one year anniversary of Winston's diagnosis. Karen and I cleared it up later, that it was actually August 28th yet, that morning, Sunday, August 25th, I woke up early and wanted to celebrate. Before church, I took Winston outside and made a short video of him fetching a ball in the yard. I turned to Facebook to share my feelings:

ONE YEAR AGO TODAY In the midst of the struggles of life... I have learned 100% that God wants to; 1. Be involved. 2. Be your comfort. 3. Show Himself mightily. 4. Save and Calm your heart. ...I relayed the story of Winston and his miraculous healing as briefly as possible. Then, I continued. .... *There are two videos here, one with Winston doing what he did up to that day.... and one from this morning, a year later... in the same yard.*

Psalm 46 tells us; 1. God is our refuge and strength, a very present help in trouble. 2. Therefore we will not fear, though the earth be removed, and though the mountains be carried to the midst of the sea; 3. Though the oceans roar and foam, though the mountains shake with their quaking. Selah. 4. There is a river, whose streams make glad the city of God, the holy place of tabernacles of the most High. 5. God is within her, she will not fall; God will help her at the break of day. 6. Nations are in uproar, kingdoms fall; He lifts His voice, the earth melts. 7. The Lord Almighty is with us; the God of Jacob is our fortress. Selah. 8. Come and see what the Lord has done, the desolations He has brought on the earth. 9. He makes wars cease to the ends of the earth. He breaks the bow and shatters the spear; He burns the chariots with fire. 10. He says, "Be still and know that I am God; I will be exalted among the nations, I will be exalted in the earth." 11. The Lord of hosts is with us; The God of Jacob is our refuge. Selah.

The responses were beautiful as people read and watched the videos. The folks who had walked this out with us for a year were going on about God's grace and miraculous hand. Then, our daughter Kaitlyn asked if I saw the one the lady wrote about a book. It was from someone I didn't know and in light of the fact that God had told me to write this book, and I was in the midst of doing so, it really got me thinking:

Heather Webster What a beautiful testimony! You should write a children's book series about Winston and his journey through cancer to build up faith in the lives of so many children who fight the cancer battle every day. What an inspiration Winston would be to them! I would go so far as to say God may want to use Winston as a therapy dog to visit hospitals to bring comfort and build up faith in those that are sick and dying. I can just see so clearly how God could use Winston to shine the light of his glory to others in need of a miracle just like

Winston! Wow! So amazing! You could title the books (Winston Wins ·
) So good! I love it! Thanks for sharing

A children's book. A children's book?? I didn't know
ANYTHING about writing a children's book, but the idea
seemed really good to me. I was intrigued to say the least but
sort of passed over it at first thinking, "I'm already writing a
book, that's the last thing I need to add to my plate."

A few days passed, and I couldn't get it out of my mind. I
wanted to know more, so I went back to my Facebook account
and looked up Heather, and sent her a private message. I
explained I knew it may have seemed strange, but would like
to talk to her about her ideas. I just wanted to know what her
thoughts were because I didn't know the first thing about
children's books. I told her she didn't have to respond, if it made
her feel strange, but I left her my phone number and asked her
to call whenever she had time. Honestly, I thought she would
think I was some kind of weirdo, and I would never hear from
her.

About a week and a half passed, and I woke up at 3 a.m.
again. I began to pray while laying in bed and my brain kicked
into overdrive. Suddenly, I could see the children's book, it's
layout, the illustrations, how I would write it involving Abby,
our youngest, working with "Winston the Wonderdog" in his
dock diving competitions. The story would be told from his
perspective and how he was healed from cancer. I could see the
whole thing. Then, something else happened. It sounds crazy,
even now as I write it, but I think I had a vision. I admit, it could
have been a dream. Honestly, I cannot say for sure, because I
know I went back to sleep at some point. Yet, it wasn't like any
dream I have had before. Either way, I could see Karen and
myself, along with Winston, in bookstores and hospital gift
shops, doing book signings. We were delivering this book, and

• the children's book, in a bundle. We were sharing and talking to children and praying with them. It was so vivid and real.

Later, as our family gathered in the kitchen, before we all went our separate ways, I excitedly shared my dream (or vision) with the girls. They all kind of looked at me as if I were losing my mind. If you ever saw the movie I referenced earlier, Close Encounters of the Third Kind, there is a moment when the dad is sitting at the table and starts building this mountain out of mashed potatoes. His wife and children are genuinely concerned, and rightfully so! Karen was looking at me like that, I think. The guy in the movie ends up building this huge mountain, from clay, in their living room, after his family leaves him. I think Karen was beginning to fear that I was about to order 1000 lbs of clay. Yet, I digress.

I was working from home that day. It was around 9:30 a.m. when I received a phone call from a number I was not familiar with. Upon answering, I was surprised to hear a woman say, "This is Heather Webster. You asked me to call you, how can I help?" I was so glad to hear from her but I did not tell her about my crazy dream/vision. I didn't want to seem that crazy! I simply explained that I wanted to pick her brain about her ideas about the children's book. I was intrigued to know what she had thought and what led her to that concept.

"Ohh, Tim, this was not just an *idea*. I clearly had a *vision from God.*" She informed me with confidence.

My brain did "the thing" that it had become used to doing. It sort of went numb with a sense of combined amazement and "you've got to be kidding me," all at once. I literally thought, "Where is this headed?"

"A vision?" I asked. "How so? Tell me about it."

"Tim, I saw you and your wife and Winston, in book stores and gift shops of hospitals all over the country doing book signings and praying with little children to be healed. Winston had on a gold cape. There were children being healed of cancer."

The term "mind blown" doesn't even touch what was happening on my end of the line. After explaining to her what God had given me, that very morning, we talked more about the book. I asked her how she found me, what brought her across my post about Winston.

"Well, a friend of yours shared it on his post, and he and I have been friends for a long time. We used to go to church together, before I moved to south Georgia. His name is John Jennings."

"Imagine that," I couldn't help but think, "A friend of John Jennings receiving visions from God. Who would have thought it?"

That afternoon I shared the entire story with my family again. Now, they were not looking at me as if I were about to start building mountains out of mashed potatoes! Abby, the "Google queen" of the house, piped up, "Hey, guess what color the ribbon is for bone cancer! Gold! And for Children's cancer, and for Canine Cancer too! All of them are Gold. Didn't she say Winston was wearing a gold cape in her vision?" Mind... Blown... Again.

Needless to say, I began working immediately on writing a children's book which in now being illustrated. Heather has been a major part of editing that book and helped me develop some ideas. It is likely, that you have obtained this book as a part of a bundle in which both works were completely suggested to me by strangers speaking on the behalf of God. How cool is that? It does take some of the pressure off of me, however, to be a good writer! I believe this has been His work of art, not mine. I hope my humanity hasn't gotten in the way of His message!

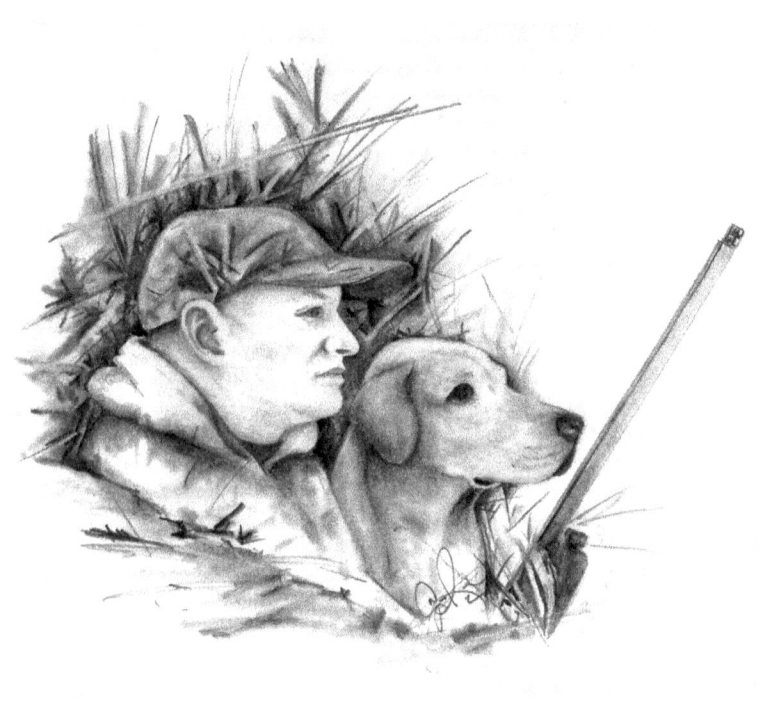

TWENTY THREE

THE RHYME AND REASON OF RANDOMNESS

Oftentimes, sickness seems to have no rhyme or reason at all. I look around me, especially at the society of cancer victims, and I almost feel like serious illness is somewhat like medieval time warfare. We watch these movies where the two armies line up on opposing hillsides. A vast valley separates them and the leaders ride their horses back and forth across the front lines shouting encouragement into their troops. When one invariably raises the courage of his men to a great enough level, the infamous trumpet sounds the signal to charge and the mass of men began to scream to the top of their lungs and run toward the front lines of the enemy. The opposing, more patient king steadfastly awaits the on-rush. He won't allow the emotional rush to dictate his actions. With careful timing, he watches the troops as they fill the valley below, running, screaming, waving their swords and shields. He glaces over his shoulder and yells at his first captain, "Archers!"

The cry carries backwards through the ranks as quickly as possible and the sound of thousands of lethal arrows fill the air overhead. The men on the front line, nervous yet filled with victorious anticipation, look up to see the arrows flying toward their foes. The sight is menacing as the arrows blacken the sky above them. There hardly seems an inch or two between them, as they soar in a mass of intended death. The oncoming soldiers continue to run forward despite the cloud of arrows that have been haphazardly flung in their direction. These arrows have not been aimed precisely. The king knows there is not an archer that can even see the oncoming army. Yet he knows, with precision, the reach of his powerful archers. He also knows of the enormous quantity of arrows with which he supplied his troops. The lethal shanks begin to descend onto the onrushing army. Many men will raise their shields and block the arrows, rendering them useless. Many arrows will simply stick into the ground, never causing any harm. Other arrows will fall lower than the edge of the shields and find their mark in the legs and lower extremities of some poor soldier, for the shields are not large enough to cover their entire bodies as they run. The attacking soldiers know, they cannot simply cower behind or below their shields for protection, they must keep up the sprint to get inside the zone where the archers can't hit them. Some of these soldiers will run through unscathed. Others will run directly into the path of a falling arrow that was launched from hundreds of yards away with no specific target intended. The arrow will find its mark past the edge of a high-held shield, coming in at just the right angle, to slip through the seam of his breastplate sinking deeply into a vital area of the running warrior. The timing of the arrow and the man have to have been absolutely perfect, yet, they are one hundred percent random. The archer in the very back who released that arrow, has no idea whether it hit its mark or not, it doesn't matter. He notches another and sends it on its way. As I watch how randomly disease befalls mankind, I can't help but think, all of us are like those running soldiers, trying desperately to get across the valley floor. The arrows of cancer, heart disease, or strokes, or virus', falling around us, finding some of us, missing others. As we make our way across the valley, the random disease strikes a friend and all we can do is keep on running as our heart breaks to watch them fall away.

In the forest, we find two lone warriors. Having made it through the initial battle, the ranks have been dispersed and scattered. The valley lay full of dead soldiers and horses. The one army over-run by the other, there are just a few men left in the woods surrounding the battlefield. The archer is hiding well as he sees his enemy sneaking into the camp of his king. The archer knows it is his moment of glory as he takes careful aim at the careless man who has begun to believe himself "untouchable." As he releases his arrow he knows the flight path was perfect. The sneaky soldier hears the wind tearing through the fletching feathers in the final moment before it arrives. The razor sharp steel of the arrowhead cuts flesh like butter and in a moment the soldier can feel his life slipping away. He had become complacent, thinking he would never get caught, thinking he would win the battle for his clan. Regardless of the injuries he had overcome in the past, regardless of how strong and fearless he had been in battle, one well placed arrow, from an unseen foe, found its mark and his life is over. Can sickness be like this as well? I want to examine two different scenarios we have in the Bible:

The first is the story from John 9 which I briefly mentioned before, from my dad's Bible study. We pick up the story in verse 2: "Who sinned and caused this man to be blind?" Jesus told them, "Neither this man nor his parents sinned," said Jesus, "but this happened so that the works of God might be displayed in

175

him." Again, I don't want to start a theological discussion about that particular statement. For this example, it's not a question of whether God *did this* or just allowed it. That is a question for another book. The point is, clearly, it was not brought on by sin. Our minds still work much like the minds of the disciples. "What did I do to deserve this?" or "How does my son deserve this?" Worst yet, "What did *I do* to cause my child to have cancer?" These are all very normal and human responses after being told someone has a life threatening disease. I believe, in many cases, it is as random as the soldiers running across the open expanse of the valley with arrows raining down on them. Obviously, there are things we can do to improve or decrease our chances of being hit. There are clear connections with life choices. For example, how we eat, if we smoke, if we drink, to use or not to use sunscreen, etc. There are so many things we can do to alter the chances of one type of sickness or another. Yet, often, some illness just appears inexplicably, regardless of how "well" we live life. So, on one side of the coin, illness seems completely random and has nothing to do with sin. The other side of this coin seems equally unfair.

In John 5:1 we read of a lame man sitting at the pool of Bethesda. According to the belief of the people there was an angel who would come down and "stir the waters" of the pools. Apparently, when the waters began to stir, the first person who slipped into the pool would be healed from whatever ailed them. I know, most of us raise our eyebrows in skepticism, thinking this must have been a local fable. However, I believe the story surrounding this pool is true. It seems unlikely, to me, that people would have stayed there, hoping to be the first person in the water, if they had not seen others being healed. In any case, there were five porches where a large number of sick people lay in wait for the waters to stir. This man had been sitting by the waters for some time, according to the scripture, and apparently, every time the waters began to stir, someone would jump ahead of him because he couldn't move, without some help. Jesus happened upon this fellow and John tells us that Jesus knew the man had been in this condition for a long time. In fact, for thirty eight years he had suffered. Jesus asked him if he wanted to be healed and of course the man began to explain his conundrum and Jesus basically told him to get up and take his bed with him. The man did so, and walked away. Jesus slipped into the crowd but later they ran into one another in the Temple. Jesus told him a very interesting thing. He said, "See, you have been made well. Sin no more, lest a worse thing come upon you." If the account in John is chronological, as it seems, this may have been the very incident which led the disciples to ask the question in John 9, concerning the blind man, and whose sin caused his illness. Upon reading this, I was shocked. I thought, "Sin no more?" You mean, like… don't sin? Ever? Or it could bring on worse condition than lying for 38 years on a mat without the ability to move? Well, who doesn't sin? I struggled, as do many, to make sense of it all. Then, I was reminded of something that Dr. Mark Rutland and his son, Travis, say often. "Jesus is speaking, 'God' and we are understanding in 'human', therefore, we may not get it." Maybe Jesus wasn't even referring to something that could happen to him during his life on earth, but rather, in the afterlife. Clearly, Jesus warned the man that he should stray from whatever it was he had in his life, or he may suffer some worse fate. However, by no means, should we link every sickness to be the result of a particular sinful life style. You may hear all kinds of spiritual hoopla over where sickness comes from and why this person got sick or whatever. If you take it back to scripture, sickness and death are rooted in satan and his intentions for mankind. I believe, this is why we see Jesus dealing with sickness in the same manner as He dealt with demons. He has compassion on its victims and simply tells it to go away. I think we waste a lot of energy and place too many hurdles before our faith by worrying about who deserves what. Jesus always healed them all. He didn't deal with who was living the right kind of life. He had compassion on the crowds of people and healed them all. He then told us all, in no uncertain terms, to do the same thing. It never mattered to Jesus where it came from. We don't have a single instance of Jesus saying, "Tell me about your family history, we may be dealing with a generational curse here." He said, "Your faith (in me) has made you whole. Go and be healthy. Live like you believe in me now." His answer was *always* the same. If you don't get anything else from reading this book, get this; If the answer is *always the same, the question doesn't matter.*[3] From a place of compassion, his answer was always, "Be healed."

It doesn't matter what the doctors say and it doesn't matter what kind of illness you are facing. It doesn't matter how serious it is or what the percentages are. I believe He wants to heal you, or your child, or your loved one, and I believe you can have faith in Him. I believe if we could stand before Him and ask Him what He thought about the mountain of sickness you face, His answer would be, "Be healed." I believe we *can* stand before Him, in spirit, and I believe His answer is still the same.

ONE FINAL QUESTION

I met a man not long ago who's wife is dying of stage 4 pancreatic cancer. I asked him if I could come pray with her and he flatly told me, "No." I asked if I could pray with him, for her and he flatly told me, "No." When I looked shocked, He said, "All my life, I have heard that Jesus is coming back. All my life, I have seen people dying around me, I have seen children being hurt by adults who were supposed to love them, I have seen people die from tsunamis, fire, car accidents. I have heard, for nearly 60 years, that God is going to do this or that. None of that has happened. We are still living in a terrible world, and all we do is destroy the world we live in and hurt each other. You can pray all you want, when you leave here, but I don't care about you praying for me or for her." I could almost feel God's heart break at his words, but I know it didn't change how God loves him. I left his store and didn't even know what to do about praying for his wife. But God knows. God loves him and his wife. God wants to heal them. Why? Because of compassion.

The final question, then, is this; Why would He heal you or your loved one? The answer is the same; God loves you, as He loves me, as He loves Hitler, as He loves Stalin, Saddam Hussein, Timothy McVeigh, Charles Manson, and my grandmother and my grandchildren. It's an impossible concept to truly grasp. Yet, it is true. In fact, it doesn't matter if you have read this book to these final words and you still sit there in unbelief. It doesn't matter if you close this book and curse me for what you think are lies or if you think I am simply misguided. It doesn't matter if you toss this book into the fireplace and curse God for giving your child cancer. It doesn't matter. Nothing changes His love for you. None of that changes His compassion for you or His desire to heal. He would heal you because He loves you. We read in the Bible; Romans 8:35-39

35 Who shall separate us from the love of Christ? Shall trouble or hardship or persecution or famine or nakedness or danger or sword? 36 As it is written: "For your sake we face death all day long; we are considered as sheep to be slaughtered."

37 No, in all these things we are more than conquerors through Him who loved us. 38 For I am convinced that neither death nor life, neither angels nor demons, neither the present nor the future, nor any powers, 39 neither height nor depth, nor anything else in all creation, will be able to separate us from the love of God that is in Christ Jesus our Lord.

One of my favorite poems I have ever read was written by Frederick Lehman:

"Could we with ink the oceans fill, and were the skies of parchment made,
were every stalk on earth a quill, and every man a scribe by trade,
To write the love of God above, would drain the oceans dry,
nor could the scroll contain the whole, tho stretched from sky to sky."

Grasp this truth. Don't let satan steal this from you. He would say to you, "Big deal, so Tim prayed for his dog and something happened, and his dog doesn't seem to have cancer anymore. Maybe the dog was misdiagnosed. So Tim prayed for his dad and then something happened and the bleeding in his heart stopped, but that was likely to happen anyway. Total coincidence! What about all the people who are praying for people who die anyway? Why do you think God would heal you or your son or your mom? Anyway, they say you have terminal cancer and there is NOTHING they can do for you at this point... who are you going to believe? This random stranger who is writing a book because he had some other random stranger say 'Habakkuk 2:2!' to him? Or are you going to believe the guys who went, for years, to school, to do this for their living?" But the answer to this question is the same as the answer to all the questions of the Gospel accounts, as was the answer to the questions of all who came before you who have seen the miraculous hand of God, the Almighty, in their lives. The answer to all the questions remains; "Be healed, in the name of Jesus, by the power of the *SAME* Spirit who raised Him from the dead, receive the fact that you are a Child of the LIVING GOD! Receive and believe that the healing for your body, or your loved one's body, was already done. By his stripes we ARE healed. Receive it, and begin thanking Him for that healing, that has ALREADY TAKEN PLACE. Be healed and forgiven. Your faith in God, be it small or great, your faith in the creator of the universe, has made you whole. Believe, with all you have, and pray that He helps your unbelief. Believe that you are loved by Him. He has compassion for you. What you have done does not matter. He WANTS to heal you so that you can tell others that you were healed BY HIM."

We won't change His love for us. And that is why He heals. Find it. Grasp it. Believe on it. Be healed.

I wanted to share with you, the reader, some photos that document this story. Some of these are not of great quality because they were taken randomly along the time this was transpiring. There are some videos as well on-line and I will provide the link to those at the bottom of these photo pages.

Be Blessed.

At the time of the most recent additions and printed edition, 4/1/2023... Winston is still doing great.

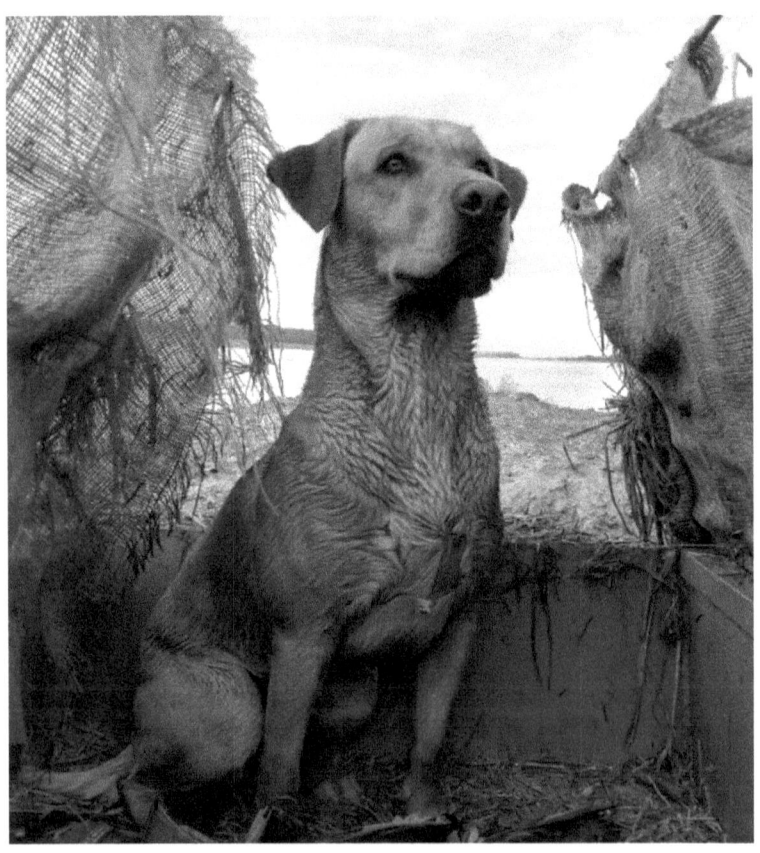

Winston in his prime 01/2018

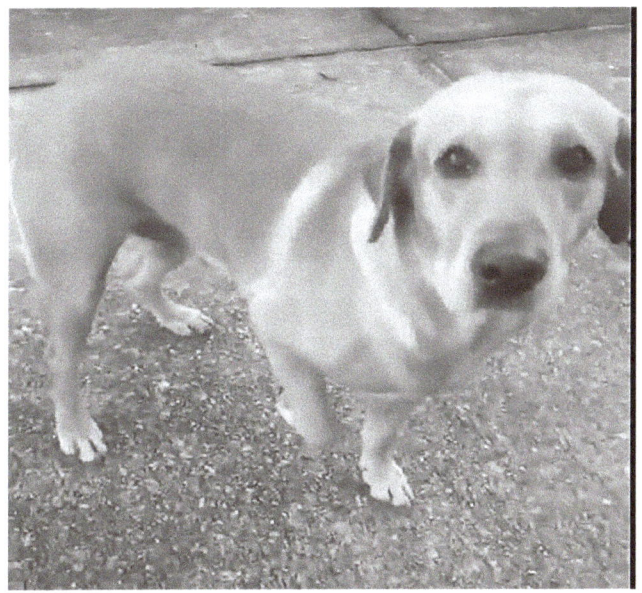

Limping 08/2018

First X-Ray 08/2018
Look closely, you can see the bone
fragmentation all around the humerus.

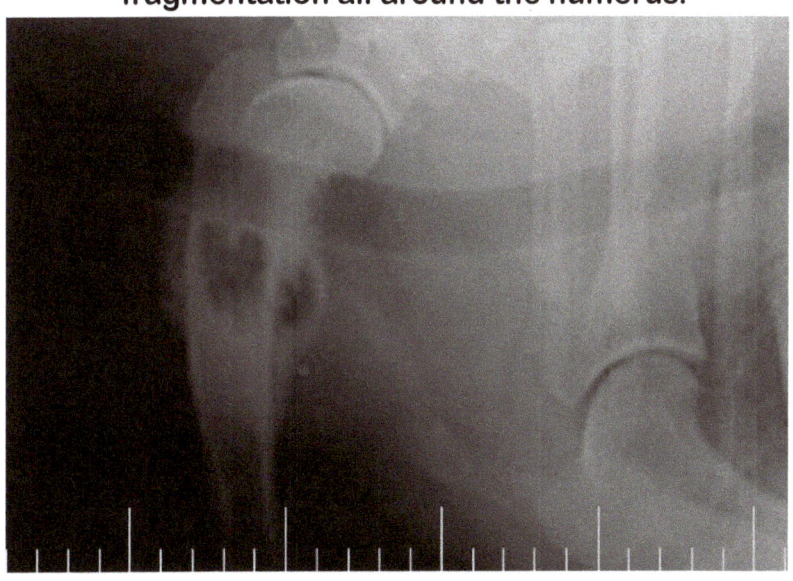

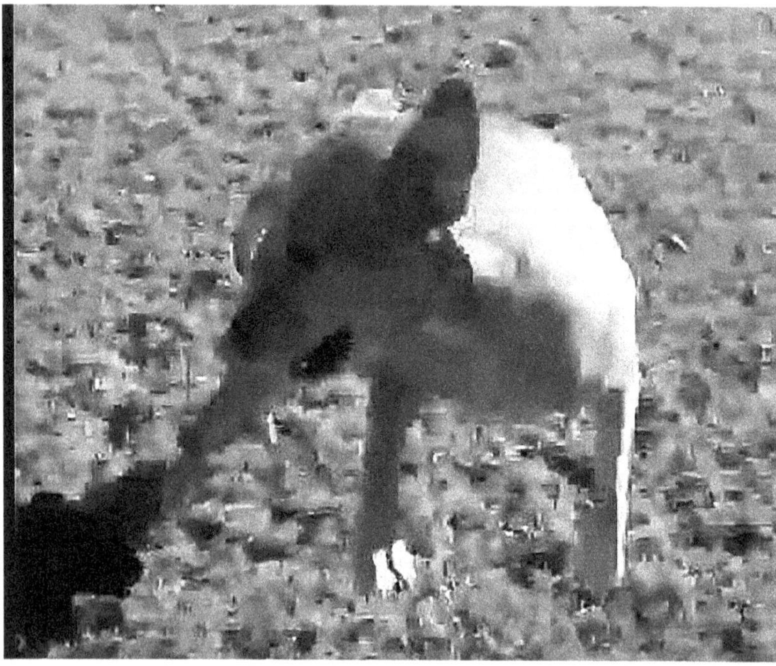

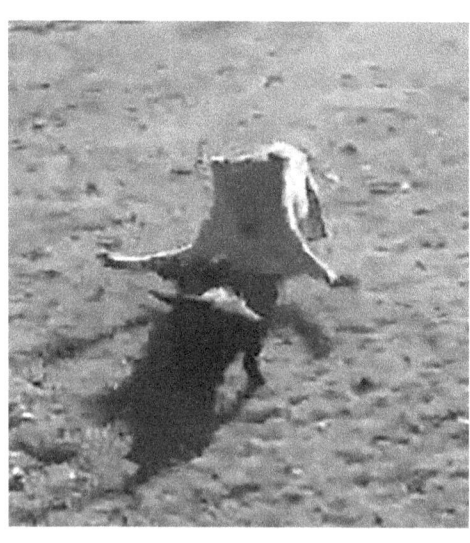

Playing with Sadie 12/09/18

Playing hard with Sadie

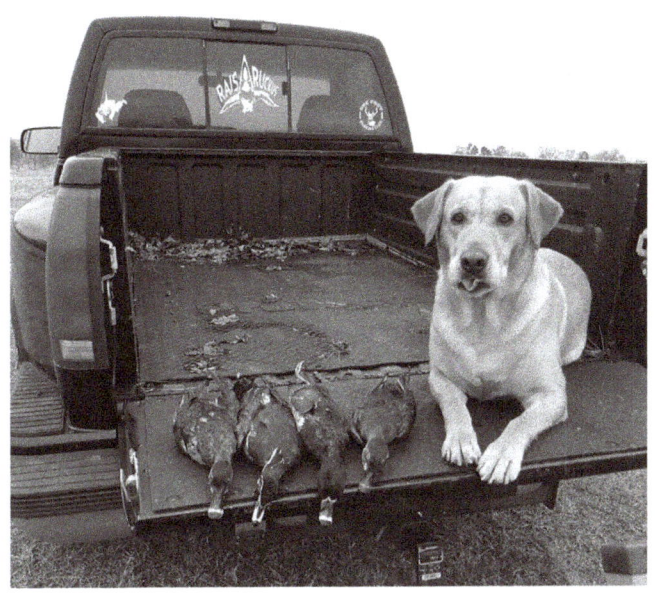

First retrieves Post Cancer12/14/18

Retrieves for young man with brain cancer 19 total 12/19/18

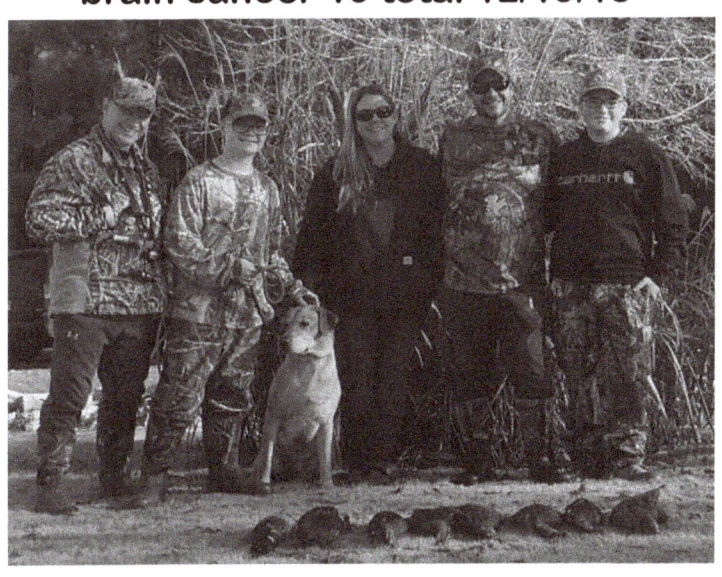

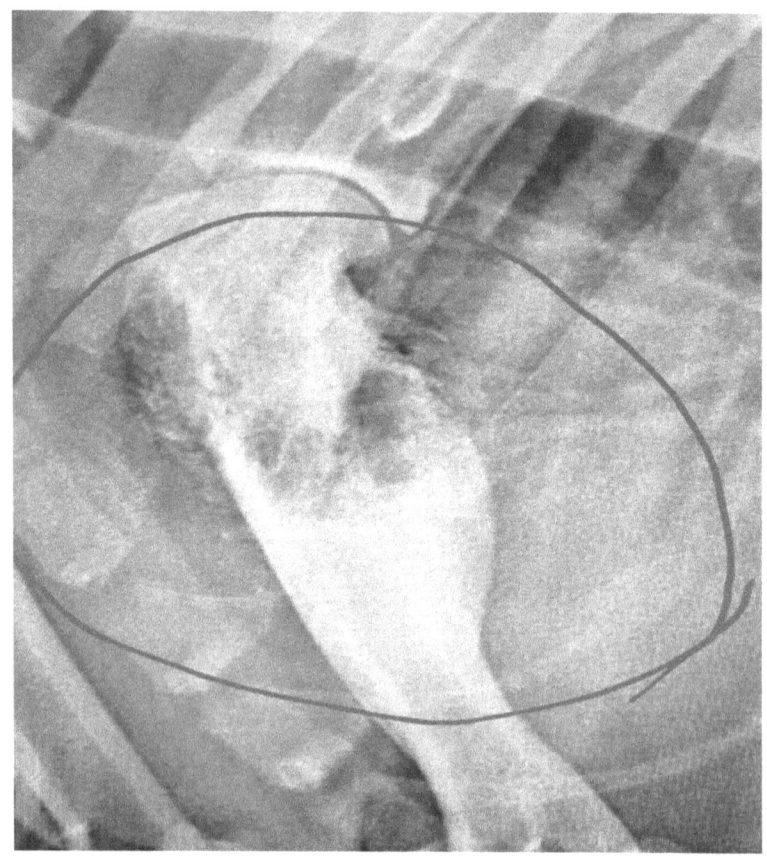

Second X-Ray 01/2019
The center of the bone appears to be closing up from top to bottom and the bone fragmentation seems to be dispersed. The obvious "hole " in the bone seems about half the size of the first x ray and the walls seem much thicker.

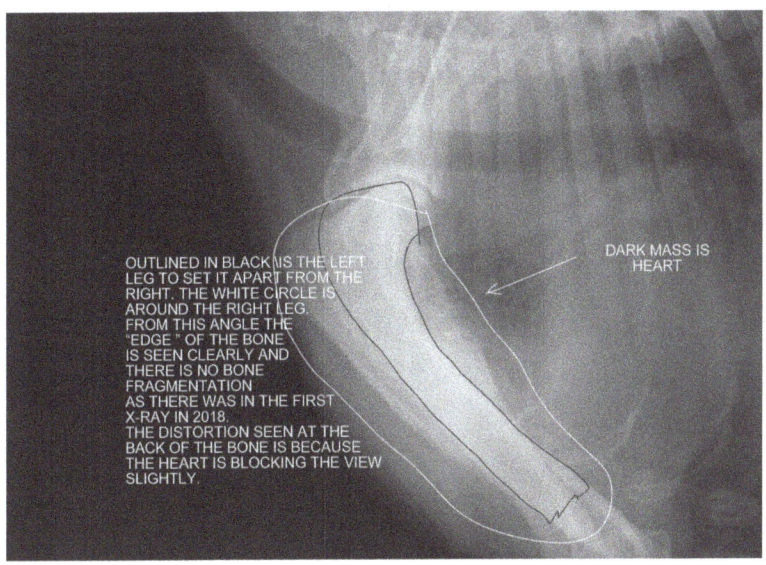

OUTLINED IN BLACK IS THE LEFT LEG TO SET IT APART FROM THE RIGHT. THE WHITE CIRCLE IS AROUND THE RIGHT LEG. FROM THIS ANGLE THE "EDGE " OF THE BONE IS SEEN CLEARLY AND THERE IS NO BONE FRAGMENTATION AS THERE WAS IN THE FIRST X-RAY IN 2018. THE DISTORTION SEEN AT THE BACK OF THE BONE IS BECAUSE THE HEART IS BLOCKING THE VIEW SLIGHTLY.

DARK MASS IS HEART

Third X-Rays 02/2022

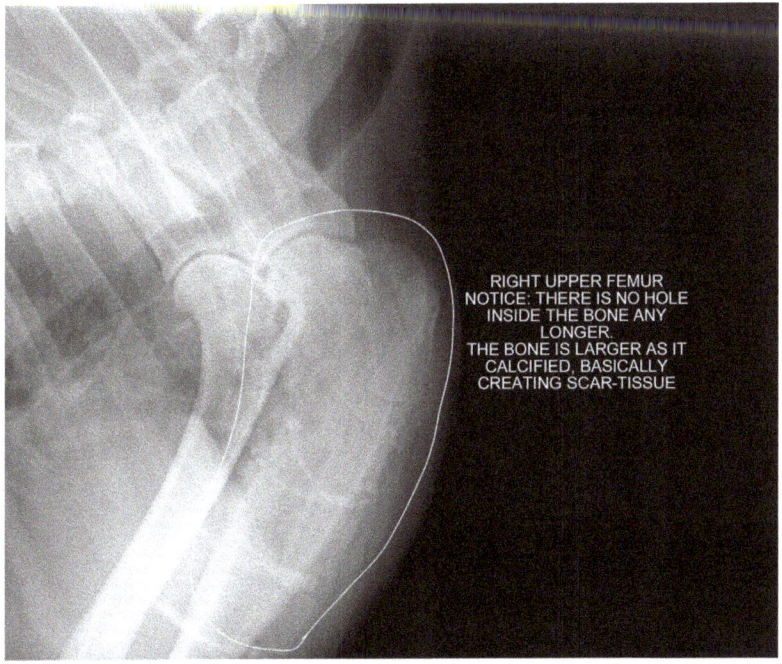

RIGHT UPPER FEMUR NOTICE: THERE IS NO HOLE INSIDE THE BONE ANY LONGER. THE BONE IS LARGER AS IT CALCIFIED, BASICALLY CREATING SCAR-TISSUE

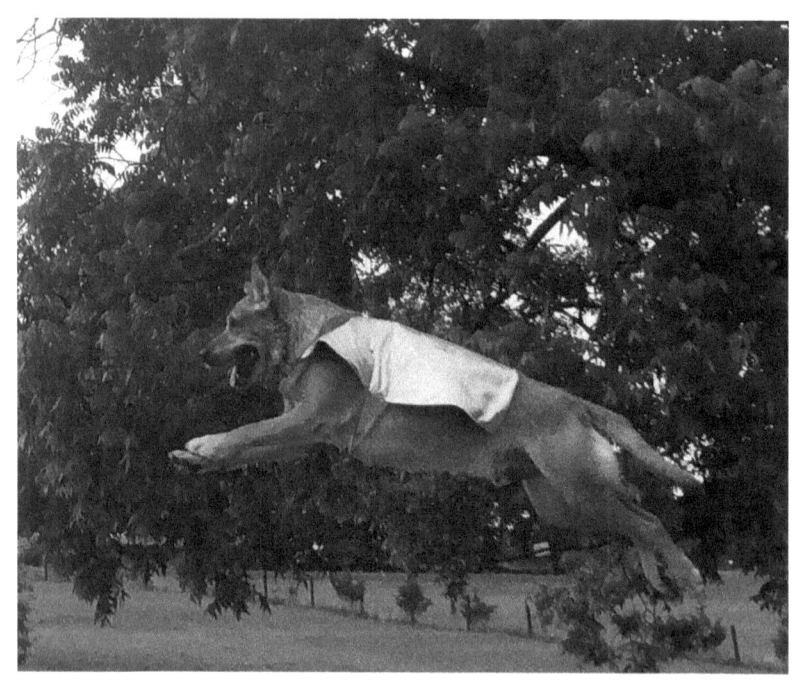

Dock Diving 04/2020
Winston doing what he loves to do.. launching himself into the water after a retrieving dummy.
Showing off his new gold cape!
His first time back at it since he was diagnosed with
bone cancer and given weeks to live, he jumped
over 18 feet!

Find Winston Videos at the following links:

Winston at 1 yr : https://youtu.be/jqJgKb4IBY0
The Story Video: https://youtu.be/Bs1ge9gNuxl

There should be more videos linked at:
www.winstonstory.com

SCRIPTURE REFERENCES:

1 John 1:9
If we confess our sins, he is faithful and just to forgive us our sins and to cleanse us from all unrighteousness.

Acts 3:19
Repent therefore, and turn again, that your sins may be blotted out.

Ephesians 1:7
In him we have redemption through his blood, the forgiveness of our trespasses, according to the riches of his grace.

Isaiah 1:18
"Come now, let us reason together," says the Lord: "though your sins are like scarlet, they shall be as white as snow; though they are red like crimson, they shall become like wool."

John 3:16
For God so loved the world, that he gave his only Son, that whoever believes in him should not perish but have eternal life.

James 5:14-15
"Is anyone among you sick? Let them call the elders of the church to pray over them and anoint them with oil in the name of the Lord. And the prayer offered in faith will make the sick person well; the Lord will raise them up. If they have sinned, they will be forgiven."

Philippians 4:19
"And my God will meet all your needs according to the riches of his glory in Christ Jesus."

James 5:1
"Therefore confess your sins to each other and pray for each other so that you may be healed. The prayer of a righteous person is powerful and effective."

Matthew 9:35
"Jesus went through all the towns and villages, teaching in their synagogues, proclaiming the good news of the kingdom and healing every disease and sickness."

Luke 6:19
"And the people all tried to touch him, because power was coming from him and healing them all."

Philippians 4:6-7
"Do not be anxious about anything, but in everything by prayer and supplication with thanksgiving let your requests be made known to God. And the peace of God, which surpasses all understanding, will guard your hearts and your minds in Christ Jesus."

1 Peter 2:24
"He himself bore our sins in his body on the tree, that we might die to sin and live to righteousness. By his wounds you have been healed."

Luke 8:50
50 Hearing this, Jesus said to Jairus, "Don't be afraid; just believe, and she will be healed."

Matthew 10:8
8 Heal the sick, raise the dead, cleanse those who have leprosy, drive out demons. Freely you have received; freely give.

Isaiah 53:4-5
Surely He has borne our griefs And carried our sorrows; Yet we esteemed Him stricken, Smitten by God, and afflicted. But He was wounded for our transgressions, He was bruised for our iniquities; The chastisement for our peace was upon Him, And by His stripes we are healed.

Matthew 21:14
Then the blind and the lame came to Him in the temple, and He healed them.

Mark 16:17-18
And these signs will follow those who believe: In My name they will cast out demons; they will speak with new tongues; they will take up serpents; and if they drink anything deadly, it will by no means hurt them; they will lay hands on the sick, and they will recover."

AUTHOR'S FINAL NOTE

1/19/25

When I first sat down to write this book, there were so many things I didn't know. One of those things was that very often, writers go back, sometimes years later, and make edits to their books. It was January 2019 when I sat down for the first time and began to explain, the best I knew how this story of God's miraculous hand. I make this edit in January of 2025. The last of many, hopefully.

In March of 2020, I wrote this:

"I have no idea how God is going to get this little book to print. These few things, I know:

Even if Winston was to take a major turn for the worse and die in a few months, God gave him back to us, for a short time, while medicine and science told us we had weeks and they were absolutely sure of their findings.

Even if the oil turns out to be fake, God used it in my life, and the lives of many others very close to me, to strengthen our faith when we had little faith.

Even if this book never goes to print and a single child never sees the Children's Book, God gave me a task, for some reason, and it has been an incredible journey working through it all."

God has seen us through all of this.. Let it be a testimony to His Miraculous hand!!

I will not bore you with all the details of the last few years, but many of those details are important for you to know. I will just say this. We have sold and/or given away over 3000 books at this point, two-plus years post the initial printing. I have revised the author's final notes 4 times. We have read the children's book to groups of students, now exceeding 1000, all over the place. We have seen the beginnings of the vision that Heather and I had of reading the book in a bookstore/ giftshop and praying for children with cancer. "Winston Wins Ministries" has become a reality and we are working on getting our 501C3 certificate and establishing a board of trustees. It has been an amazing 2 years and I am looking forward to seeing what God is going to do with all of this. But first, let's talk about some things that happened over the last six years.

Two things happened that have served as an attack on my confidence. Remember, satan wants our faith to be shaken, the last thing he wants is for us to be able to stand in confident faith, in the face of his attacks on our lives. Clearly, these two things were not only about attacking me, for they were both much, much larger in the grand scheme of things. Yet, they both rattled me. After much thought, I felt I could not ignore them and simply dismiss them from the book, at least as an afterthought.

In chapter 6 I told you about a possible miracle that involved oil. I am very aware that there is a lot of negative press about this oil. I cannot, in good conscience, tell you that I know the whole truth about it. I only know what my experiences were with the people involved and with the oil. Assuming you have read the whole book, then you know that this story does not say that we poured oil on my dog and he was instantly healed. If you are here, skipping ahead, I will say here and now, that is not what happened.

If you stop here and go and research the oil, and choose

then not to finish the book, you will have done yourself a great disservice. It would be the epitome of throwing out the baby with the bathwater, as they say. So, I want to be clear, because I have now experienced this first-hand, you are going to question the validity of the information contained in chapter 6 and you will go to the internet and research it and you will find all the ugliness of the world there. To be honest, I had my own doubts about all of this in the beginning, as well.

This is what I know. We are all broken vessels. God uses broken vessels in many, many great ways. Therefore, we cannot allow the eventual sinful breakdown of people to undermine the incredible hand of God on those same people at a given time. I have led people to the Lord and baptized people over the years. And then I sinned. Does my eventual sin negate their salvation? By no means! If that were the case, then all the people saved in a crusade held by a famous pastor in the '70s and '80s who then fell to sin and destroyed his ministry, would have to go back and find the Lord all over again! It's a ridiculous thought. I said all of that to say this;

The human, sinful nature that eventually exemplifies the weakness of a man does, in no way, negate God's ability to use that man in an incredible way. Nor does it negate the effect on people's lives that God has while using that man. It does not even keep God from restoring and using that man again! I'm guessing that David and his actions that resulted from his rooftop exploits and his murderous behavior would have had all of us questioning whether or not he was a very Godly man. Then God used the exact same couple to bring forth Solomon. We need to be cautious with how we simply write people off for their poor decisions. Glass houses and stones and all that.

Every single word I have written in this book is true to my knowledge. I have made great efforts to be as truthful as possible with you and to tell this story with as much genuine transparency as I could muster. We were not associated with the bookstore or the persons who owned it or the Bible. We became affiliated by friendship alone. To this day, I cannot tell you if the entire thing was a scam or not. I believe Johnny when he says it was not. But there is no way for me to verify that. I know a few things about it; I know what God told me about it. I know what He told me to do with it and I know what happened. The oil, for us, became a small part of a much larger picture. I could have chosen to cut it all out. But I believe I am not supposed to and I believe I know why.

There are a few very strong lessons to learn here; 1. God can do miracles with whatever/whomever He chooses to use, even if it's someone's attempt at deceiving the world. 2. We should ALWAYS give God the glory and never try to rob Him of that. 3. When God promises something, we can have faith in that. He does not need our help in accomplishing the supernatural. 4. The two main ingredients in seeing God work in and through our lives, are faith and obedience.

If you are like most people who read this book, you have already gotten on your device and researched the oil and you have already read the world's opinion of how that all went down. I would like to discuss this here and share with you some points that you would have otherwise been incapable of knowing unless you know the people from there as I do now. I have spoken with Johnny and he has given me permission to discuss this at length in my book so here goes:

There is a newspaper writer from Chattanooga, Tennessee who was doing a story on the oil in Dalton. His first writing about the ministry and the oil seemed ambiguous enough, only mildly shaded, in my opinion, towards skepticism. (Fair enough) Afterward, the writer allegedly received a tip from someone in Dalton, stating that they had seen Jerry, (the owner of the Bible that leaks oil) in a local store buying mineral oil.

This, apparently, happened in the fall of 2019. The writer then drove down to Dalton and went into the local store and asked a couple of managers if they could corroborate the tip. (It is unknown if one of them was the original "tipper" to begin with.) The managers claimed they had seen Jerry in the store, buying a large amount of mineral oil. The writer then, in January of 2020, made an addition to his original story and planned to have some of the oil from the Bible tested by the chemistry department of the local university. According to the final article released by the newspaper, the oil was a very close match to the mineral oil supplied by the store. To make things more suspicious, the Bible quit producing oil in January 2020.

I spoke with Johnny concerning this and he informed me Jerry admitted, that at one point, the Bible had quit producing oil and he had gone to the store in question, purchased mineral oil, and had intended on mixing it into the oil, in his words, "To help God." He admitted it was a horrible thing to think of doing and has expressed his greatest sorrow over caving to the temptation. However, he claimed at that point he never put it in the container with the Bible. Johnny had several vials of the oil lying around in his office that were collected from the beginning, as well as access to many vials collected throughout the time of the ministry's lifespan. He sent several of these to be tested based on their dates of collection.

Covid then took over the world. After some time I spoke with Johnny again. The shutdown slowed this process greatly. His findings were the oil that was collected early on, until around the Fall of 2019, tested the same as it had before; Impossible to determine exactly what it was, yet it didn't have any man-made material.

However, the oil collected around the winter - spring of 2019-2020, had Mineral oil in it. So, Jerry lied. He had put some mineral oil in the container. For exactly how long it is unknown.

We do know that the content of the oil changed considerably near the end of 2019. You will not read that part in the news or likely on the internet. They do not want to credit God with the miraculous. They only want to tear down what they do not understand.

Here's my take. At this point, I don't care. I know that sounds intentionally blind. But, here's the deal….

God TOLD me clearly, "The oil is just oil, it is something physical to hang your faith on. It is your faith (in ME) that heals!" Also, I don't care about what they found, because I KNOW what happened in my life, surrounding the oil. If Jerry was a fake, and I do not believe he originally was, but if he was, God used the oil and the testimony of many people to bring about many things with which I have a personal connection. I could write a small book on the things that I or someone very close to me, experienced in connection to the oil! All inexplicable by the laws of nature. God used the oil in our lives, to help us build our faith. If it was a hoax the entire time, then, shame on them, but let all glory and honor and praise be to God who can even turn a hoax into a blessing! If it was fake the entire time, then God used a satanically designed hoax to create miracles from it! Which one is more miraculous? Oil coming from a Bible that seems to have miraculous power or oil poured over a Bible by a man in need of attention, that still played a part in the miraculous healing of people and animals?

I want to remind you of the story of Abraham and Sarah that I wrote of years ago in this book. They heard from God about Isaac. God told them they would have a son. In a moment of weakness, Sarah decided to "help God" fulfill His plan. When she sent Abraham into the tent with her maidservant, all she was doing was the exact thing Jerry did. In a moment of fear and doubt, she turned to her own solution for the problem. I truly, truly believe that the Bible was at one point, genuinely leaking oil, and that oil was a miracle by God, to help people with their faith. Jerry, at some point, feeling like it was something that "just couldn't stop" bought oil and added it to what was in the container. He fell prey to the same temptation Abraham did. How rough can we be on a person who was tempted by the same sin as the Father of the Nation of Israel?

Another noteworthy point is this; After hearing all of this Karen and I went to the shelf and pulled down some mineral oil. (We had it in a basket on a shelf for some reason, which I do not remember) We compared it to our own bottle of "Bible Oil" as scientifically as we could! We felt them both with our fingers, no comparison! We smelled them both, the mineral oil has a very distinct smell and the Bible Oil does not. I even tasted them. The Mineral Oil was unpleasant. The Bible Oil had no taste at all. I am not sure what he did to the mineral oil to make it so much smoother, less smelly, and remove the taste, but if Jerry put mineral oil in the oil I have, I certainly could not tell! One more "scientific test; Winston will lap the Bible Oil from my hand like it is sugar water. He would not lick the mineral oil for whatever reason.

The sad truth is we are all human and all tempted in different ways. Deceit is an ugly sin, of which we are all guilty. There is not a human alive who has not, at one time or another, told a lie. I admit, to lie about something like this is considerably grievous. Yet, I can empathize with his fear of the oil running dry and the ministry grinding to a halt. Obviously, we can all stand in judgment and say, "That is exactly what he should have done!" I agree. I am sure, in retrospect, he would agree. The most amazing thing about God's Grace and Mercy is that it is for all of us, no matter what we have done. Even lying about a miraculous event to further push along a ministry that has done great things.

The saddest part of all of this was the latest news I received concerning it. Jerry went home and shut out the world. In his grief, and shame I assume, he refused to come back to church. I do not know how the people of that area treated him. I cannot attest to any of that. I cannot imagine the feeling of knowing that the entire world around you knows your darkest sin of deceiving people and tearing down something that God had done. The regret, I imagine, was huge. He sat in his house refusing to be restored to his community, got sick, and died. I suppose there may be more to the story there. I do not know of any other details. I simply know that he passed away and it breaks my heart. The bookstore has now been sold and new beginnings have happened to all the people I got to know from there. Amazingly, I still have about 4 vials of oil sitting on my bookshelf and I do not hesitate to anoint someone with it for prayer. Winston still laps it up as if it were steak drippings. One day, maybe, we will know all there is to know about the oil that came from Jerry's bible. For now, I know all I need to know.

I know what the oil did in my life and I saw miracles surrounding the use of it in other's lives. I also know what God told me about it, and I have seen miracles of healing without it. I don't know why things happen the way they do and all I can do is tell you my story. That is what I have attempted to do. You are faced with a crossroads of sorts here: You can believe what I have said and believe that it was, at one point, a miracle, or you can choose to not believe at all. Your belief has absolutely no effect on its truthfulness. My story is either true, or I (and a lot of other people) am crazy, or I am a liar. You have to choose at this point, for yourself, how you are going to receive this and move on.

The second thing which happened rattled me even more. Dewitt, the wonderful gentleman who spoke words over us and basically told me God wanted me to write this book, went to be with the Lord in March 2020. Despite our prayers and faith and pleading and anointing him with oil and fasting, he passed away, having suffered a brain bleed. My heart sank into deep depths of sadness over his passing, and then, God asked me, "Are you just going to sulk or are you going to get back to doing what I told you to do? He is mine now, I have him."

I do not pretend to understand all of the "whys and hows" of this life, this world, this faith, our God, His sovereign will, and all of that. I believe I will understand more fully one day. I believe God is on the throne and I believe He loves us, both you and me. I believe His will is for us to be healthy until He calls us home. I believe the Bible is His Word to man and we can lean on it, and follow it, and have faith in the Word of God.

UP TO DATE WITH WINSTON

Remember they told us the bone would be super-fragile? Well, we built a new house three years ago and during construction, he was upstairs with Abby, I walked out of the front door talking to a subcontractor, and Winston decided to come to me the most direct way possible. He jumped out of the window onto the roof over the front porch and jumped off the roof. It scared us all to death, as you can imagine, but he was perfectly fine. I am guessing the bone is not so fragile. That was in the late summer of 2020.

Back on 02/09/22, I made this entry in my journal:

Winston got up from his bed three days ago limping on the other foot. One of the things the vets had told me was that the cancer would move from leg to leg. I had been playing with him in the yard that afternoon and he had been fetching very hard, yet, to see him limping and not have a visible reason for it scared me to death. I massaged his left shoulder and gave him a Tylenol. The next morning…still limping. I called my friend, the chiropractor, "Could we x-ray Winston again?"

We had actually been saying for 3 years we wanted to anyway. That morning, we met before his office opened. I have attached the photo of the x-ray. You can see in the photo that the upper portion of his right humerus is enlarged but the hole that was there is completely gone. The reason the bone looks a little fuzzy is because it is in the foreground of the picture. It is the best shot we got of the right leg, while actually trying to x-ray the left leg. The left leg, by the way, looks perfectly fine. We are convinced it was a strain of some sort and he is fully recovered now.

Here is that x-ray.

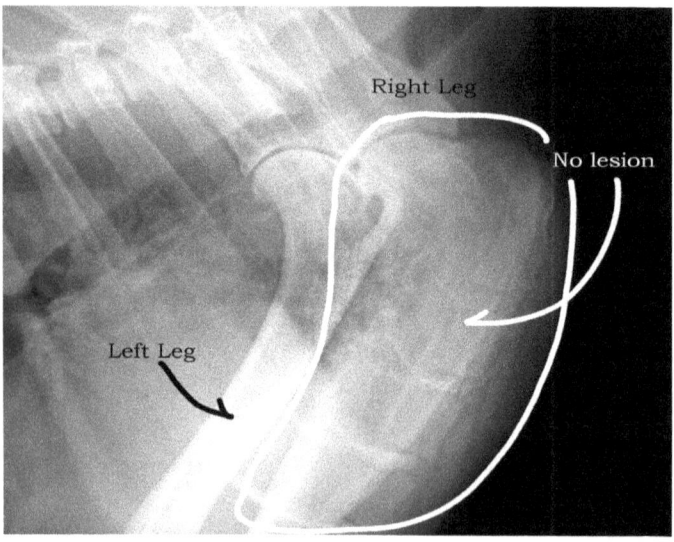

At the writing of this, my dog lays at my feet and snores and we are 6 + years from when Winston was diagnosed. He is as strong as ever, if not stronger. In the spring of 2023, we were invited to go to a Veterinarian conference with a company I have become acquainted with, Pet-Genex. An advantage of having been at the vet conference was we had a huge concentration of veterinarians there who didn't have anything to prove about this case. We had a very interesting visit with one particular vet who was seemingly a non-Christian, possibly an atheist, and a bone specialist. She saw our images of Winston's latest x-ray compared to the first one. She explained that both cancer and a particular fungal infection can present this way in the bone. Both conditions destroy the cells that make osteoblast. Osteoblast is required for the rebuilding or "remodeling" of bone. It is how a broken bone is bonded back when healing. It usually causes something called hypertrophy which is why Winston's bone is larger than normal even now. You can see it in the x-ray image. If you go back through all the images we have included you see the hypertrophy is getting better and better. In this particular x-ray, you can also see how solid the bone is. That is referred to as hypertrophic remodeling. This is what was simply astonishing to the bone specialist veterinarian. She stood there trying to take it all in and then asked for a copy of my book. She said it simply does not happen with bone cancer or with the fungal infection she had mentioned. She said the cells involved will have lost their ability to create the necessary osteoblast required for remodeling. All I can say is.... "but God...."

At the conference, we were introduced to The Christian Vet Mission (CVA). They combine mission work with Vet services and do great work all over the world. We began talking about speaking at one of their weekend retreats where I would get to share Winston's story with vet students and vets from the local area at UGA's veterinarian school. After hours of discussion, my contact with CVA suggested that we visit the vet medical center, with Winston, for an official report from their board-certified radiologist about Winston's original condition and his present condition. Her feelings were "If we were going to be speaking to a scientific community like vet students, we would need this to provide more validity in the minds of those attending the presentation." So, we went to the UGA Vet Med Center on 8/14/23 to do just that. I have included all the images for comparison from the beginning to the end and a layperson's (me) summary of the report from the radiologist. If you would like to have a copy of the actual radiologist's report that speaks in a completely different language than I do, email me.

On 8/22/23 I finally spoke with the veterinary student from UGA Vet Med Center and she translated the radiologist report into layman's language for me. I will summarize that 50-minute conversation here. First, let me say that the radiologist cannot and will not attempt to diagnose any particular illness from radiographs alone. Their job is to read, as accurately as possible, the radiograph and attempt to decipher what they see. Let me add that it is impossible to remove the human factor.

The radiologist, as well as the vets who saw Winston on 8/14/23, was viewing all of this through this perspective; We are looking at a dog 5 years post-diagnosis, alive and well, with a bone that is still in the process of healing. If God is not in the equation, if a miracle is not a possibility, then their perspective would be that all the vets that viewed his x-rays in 2018 were possibly too quick to call his condition "Osteosarcoma" which is terminal, malignant bone cancer. Through the lens of "the dog is walking around and seemingly healed" this is a reasonable conclusion because there are, according to the radiologist's report, a number of different things that could present, on an X-ray, like the x-ray from 2018; There are fungal infections, there are reactions to severe bone trauma, and there are other types of bone cancer that are benign. There is simply no way to know for sure, without a bone biopsy, to know if the cells inside the bone contain malignant cancer. The vet admitted that those cells may or may not be present now considering the level of repair the bone has undergone.

The only way to be sure was to perform a biopsy much sooner, maybe in 2018. Of course, everyone agrees, at that point, given the limited perspective they had in 2018, they were indicating he had weeks to live without very expensive, aggressive treatment for the bone cancer. (of which they were all very sure he had)

So, let's take a look back at who was this "they" that I am talking about. Who is included in the team of vets who diagnosed him to the best of their ability through the radiographs they had. The attending vet in 2018 had years of experience and her own practice. She was very clear about her diagnosis. However, she did tell me to be 100% sure about it they could perform some other tests (I assume a bone biopsy) but she said, "I can just tell you, that's bone cancer. I have seen it many times and this is where it usually presents itself in large dogs." I remember that statement.I then sent pictures of those x-rays to my friend Keith who had been a vet in my life for over 20 years. He had owned his own practice for years and was the most no-nonsense, never- jump-to-conclusions, vet I have ever worked with. He was also a good friend of mine and a strong Christian. I literally texted him and said I thought the vet I was seeing had lost her mind. I said, "She says he has bone cancer and that he is likely going to die!" Keith told me, "I am sorry buddy. I would have to agree with her and you are in a tough spot. I hate to tell you this, I am sorry." It was only after Keith said that to me that the reality of it all began to settle in on me.

Third, was the attending vet's "good friend" who was supposedly the "Head of the Oncology Department at UGA Vet School." The HEAD of the CANCER Department looked at these images and agreed that he had osteosarcoma.

Fourth, and a week or so later, was my own mobile vet. She agreed with the diagnosis and began to work with us to create a plan not only for living with this terminal cancer patient but for end-of-life considerations. She explained in great detail the fragility of the bone and through her, I purchased the shots for dealing with WHEN the bone finally gave way. Not IF, but WHEN.

The attending vet was so convinced that this was terminal cancer, she was willing to remove the leg, up to the ball joint, the VERY NEXT DAY. (To the tune of $4,000.00 and would give us about 4 months with him)...When I asked her, "What would you do?" She flatly exclaimed, "I would be in my car taking my dog to the University to begin chemotherapy treatment." (She explained that would be between $10-12,000.00 and would give us about a year with him.)

Finally, I had the bone specialist at the vet conference who told me, "There could be a few other things that presented like his original x-rays that were not bone cancer, but, given his sudden onset of lameness, the location of the lesion, and the lack of any accompanying symptoms, I would have to agree that it was likely osteosarcoma. Although, even if it wasn't, the other things would not have healed the way it was healing and the bone would have not had the ability for hypertrophic remodeling." (the rebuilding of bone through osteoblast, a cellular "welding" agent that repairs broken bones, etc) She explained that the cells that create osteoblast would have died under all the conditions that would present like this on a radiograph.

Clearly, through the perspective they all had, Winston had malignant osteosarcoma and it was very advanced and we had very little time with him. Clearly, through the perspective we all had, there was little reason to spend the money on a battery of tests to rule out terminal bone cancer. Clearly, I knew what God said to me and knew there was no reason to go through any more tests. I bet Winston's life on faith that I had heard God say he was going to be ok. I honored God by proclaiming it in front of the vet and her staff and then to everyone who would lend me their ear. I never thought we would be here, starting a ministry, reading books to children, and giving talks to adults and vet students. I never thought for a second we would be forming a board and applying for a 501(c)(3). I just knew what a lot of very qualified people told me about my dog, I also knew what God said to me about my dog.

The vets at UGA, in my opinion, are at a disadvantage because they can essentially see the end of the story and that has an effect on the narrative they would use to give their opinions about the beginning of the story. Even a believer has to use caution, simply because of human skepticism, in saying they can look back at those x-rays and know that it was malignant bone cancer. They are right to some degree. They, and therefore we, cannot know, beyond a shadow of a doubt, that it was correctly diagnosed by 3 well-seasoned vets and the head of the oncology department of their own school. However, even the vet who discussed this with me claimed, "This does not take away from the miraculous healing aspect of this by any means. All the things that are described as possible reasons for the lesions on his bone would have required aggressive medical treatment, and all you did was take him home and pray over him and anoint him with oil and all of those things are pretty much better." I say "pretty much better" because there is something that still bothers them about the radio-graphs of Winston's leg. Look closely. the outside edges of the bone are fuzzy. You can see some type of material surrounding the bone. They told me it was Periosteal Proliferation. That is a fancy way of saying the cellular tissue that surrounds the bone is expanded in order to protect the bone because it has suffered some kind of trauma. I asked if that meant "scar tissue" and the vet said, "In a sense, yes." So, what I was told was possibly bone fragmentation floating out from the bone is actually Periosteal Proliferation, the bone's own way of protecting itself. It must do a pretty good job... remember, 3 years ago he jumped off my roof and landed on all fours... I guess the bone wasn't as fragile as it should have been! Praise the Lord!!!

I have included this long-winded Author's note to be as transparent and honest with my readers as possible. I have gone down all the rabbit holes and side trails to give you the best view of this story I can. Am I slightly biased? Sure I am. Do I believe that Winston had terminal, malignant, Osteosarcoma that should have killed him in a few weeks? I sure do. I trust in the expertise of the vets who saw him in 2018. I trust the opinions of the Head of the Oncology Department at UGA Vet School and the Bone Specialist at the conference. 3 of the 5 of them had absolutely nothing to gain by giving me their utmost honest opinion. In fact, the bone specialist all but told me that she was an atheist. Her statements were confusing to herself and she seemed to barely believe that she was seeing the same dog and that all we had done was pray over him. She said, "This doesn't happen!" Then told me why it "doesn't happen" and then said she needed to read the book... she was simply astounded.

I don't discredit the vets at UGA. They were fantastic with Winston and have spent a LOT of time discussing all of this with me and, in my opinion, have been extremely forthcoming, sensitive, and open to all avenues of discussion. I simply believe they are stuck. They do not have enough evidence to confidently diagnose or rule out anything. They are stuck here in 2023 without the ability to erase from their perspective that the dog outlived the original diagnosis. They see some kind of issues still surrounding his bone and all of it leads to saying, "We cannot diagnose nor can we rule out anything at this point."

Some people may believe that Winston should not have had any issues surrounding his bone if God had actually healed him. I can see their point... but in that line of thinking, let me pose this question; Shouldn't Jesus' hands have been completely healed after he was raised from the dead? They were not according to John. John 20:24-30: Thomas (called

Didymus) was one of the twelve, but he was not with the other followers when Jesus came. They told him, "We saw the Lord." Thomas said, "That's hard to believe. I will have to see the nail holes in his hands, put my finger where the nails were, and put my hand into his side. Only then will I believe it." A week later the followers were in the house again, and Thomas was with them. The doors were locked, but Jesus came and stood among them. He said, "Peace be with you!" Then he said to Thomas, "Put your finger here. Look at my hands. Put your hand here in my side. Stop doubting and believe." Thomas said to Jesus, "My Lord and my God!" Jesus said to him, "You believe because you see me. Great blessings belong to the people who believe without seeing me!"

I can understand Thomas' reluctance to believe that Jesus was alive again. I understand the lack of faith in many because I have suffered too with that lack of faith. I have doubted many times if it was all real. I have questioned my own faith and the validity of stories like this one. I have stood outside at night staring up at all those stars and felt insignificant, tiny and so temporary. I have wondered if our existence was meaningless and if there was a God and if so, where was He in all of this chaos? I have wondered why He would show up for some and not for others. I have thought about how I would do it differently if He asked me how it should be done. I have controverted over the outcome of many catastrophes and speculated about how I thought He should have done things. I would not have saved a guy's dog and let a mother's daughter die from cancer at the same time. Yet, He is God. His ways are higher than mine.

One more thing. Our middle daughter got married. She married a great guy who is serving in the military and he was stationed in Texas. She moved to Texas and while he was in South Korea she was alone in Texas for several months.

Sadie, "my Ishmael" moved with her and served as her source of sanity while she lived alone. They are quite the pair. Had it not been for Sadie I don't know what she would have done. Had we never lost Heidi, Sadie wouldn't have come. Had Winston not had cancer, Sadie would not have come. My wife would never have let Heidi go with our daughter Katy... God has His ways of using all things for our good. Hmm. Sounds familiar. Romans 8:28.

I no longer pontificate about how He does things. God's thoughts are above my thoughts. I am hyper-conscious of this; He has shown grace and mercy to me when I did not deserve it. He loves me and He loves you beyond our comprehension. What is important to me, is important to Him, and our faith, or the lack of our faith, has no bearing on His existence or His faithfulness. If you choose to believe this story or if you write it off as the memoirs of a lunatic, that has no effect on its authenticity.

As I attempt to finish this, I reflect on the last six years. We have quarantined at home from the corona virus. We have seen political shake ups. We have watched the country and the world turns itself on its head and have seen some of the greatest levels of confusion I can remember. The entire world is in an up-roar over finances, people dying, a shortage of essential goods, and political issues that have nothing to do with any of this. Trust in the government is at an all time low. Trust in institutions as a whole seems to have diminished. There have been riots, and social outrage is at a level I don't recall in my life. I have no idea what the future holds, be it the immediate future, or the long term future. What I am sure of is we can trust God. We can trust His word. He is in our corner even when it doesn't feel like it. He is watching over us and although we may face uncertainty and trials and pain, He promises that if we love him, we can count on ALL things working together for our good. ALL THINGS! I believe it is in His plan for you to do so, and I believe He wants to work a miracle in your life!

208

God is sovereign. We can stamp our feet and do all the things "right" and demand sickness to do this or that, and occasionally, God's answer will be "No." We will understand it all on the other side of Heaven's door, I believe.

God is still working miracles, and if you are reading this, then I believe it is in His plan for you, and I believe He wants to work a miracle in your life!

Folks, this has been a long, stretched-out story, that spanned a lot of time. I pray that I have done what He meant when he sent Dewitt over to my table to yell, "Habakkuk 2:2!" at me. (Then the LORD replied: "Write down the revelation and make it plain on tablets so that a herald may run with it.) I pray that this book has accomplished what it was supposed to accomplish. Finally, I pray you have been blessed by the time you spent with us. I want to tell you how much I appreciate you taking this journey with my family, Winston, and me.

Meanwhile, I pray now, that the words given to me by the Holy Spirit, that fill the pages before this one, fall on hearts and minds that need to hear them. I pray those words bring peace and soothing to hurting spirits. I pray that God uses even the likes of me, in your life, to lift you to a new faith in Him. I pray that you find Him, His peace and His rest in what you have read. And, I pray that in the name of Jesus, you are healed.

Thank you for allowing me to tell you The Winston Story.
Tim A. Rupard

God is good. He is sovereign. His will is for us to be healthy and live in victory. I believe we can. I want you to be able to reach out to us if you want prayer for healing. I may regret this, but my email for this is gooddogreads@gmail.com.

Be Blessed.
Tim Rupard

The video link to watch a quick video of Winston, Heidi and Sadie is here: https://youtu.be/h5Rg1lDdQZw

In case it has changed locations go to the main channel here and you should find all his videos. https://www.youtube.com/channel/UC6883e6TisPIRmavZO77_ag

The official Winston Video

Wincy Wins YT Channel

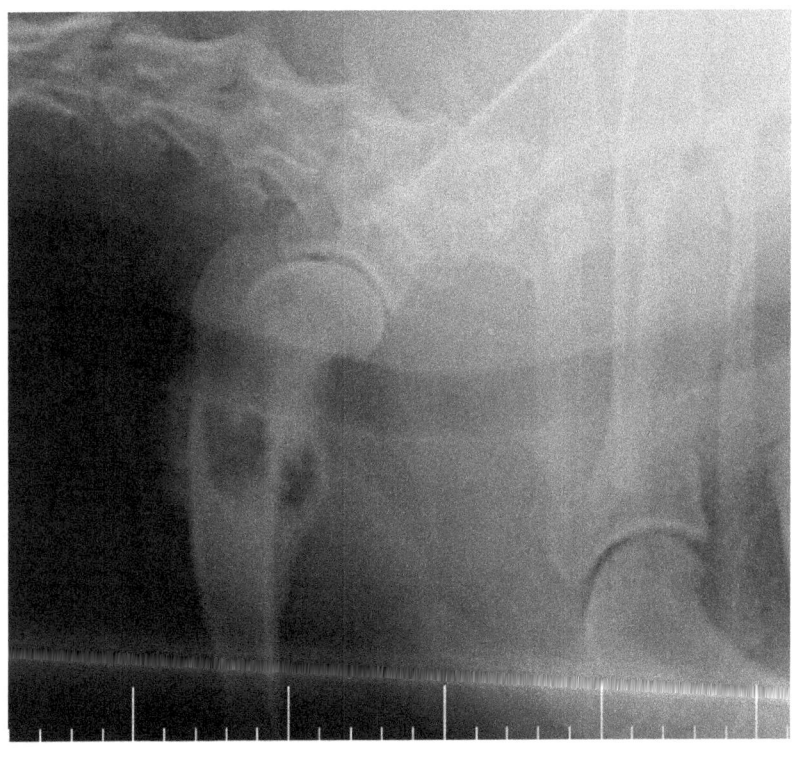

Original xray 8/22/2018 with cancer

Following are the xray images from 2018 until 2023

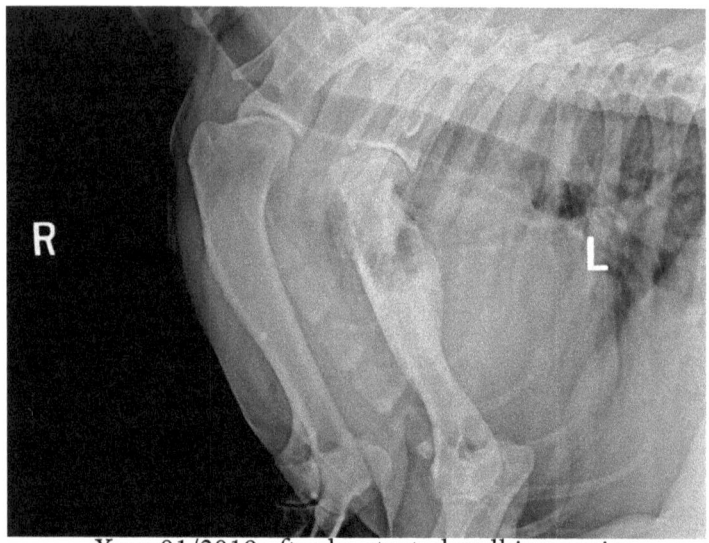

Xray 01/2019 after he started walking again showing the hole beginning to close up

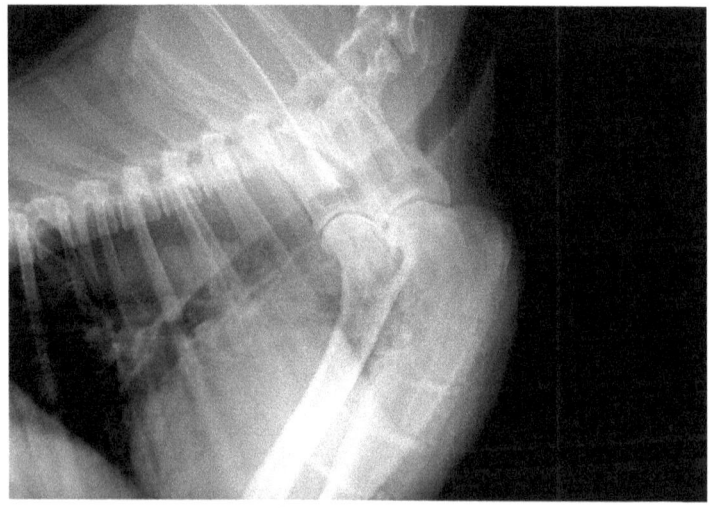

Xray 02/2022 The hole is gone, hypertrophic remodeling has occurred but still showing an enlarged bone.

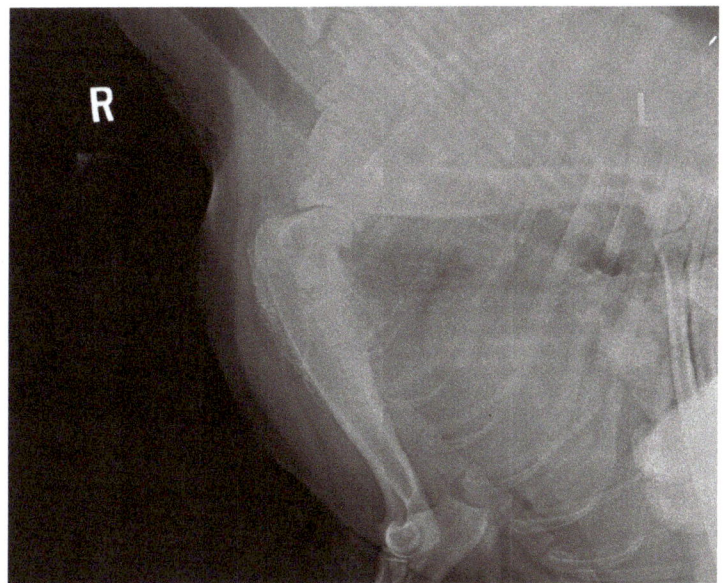

Winston's xray 3/21/2023 with no cancer. Obvious hypertrophy yet with total hypertrophic remodeling

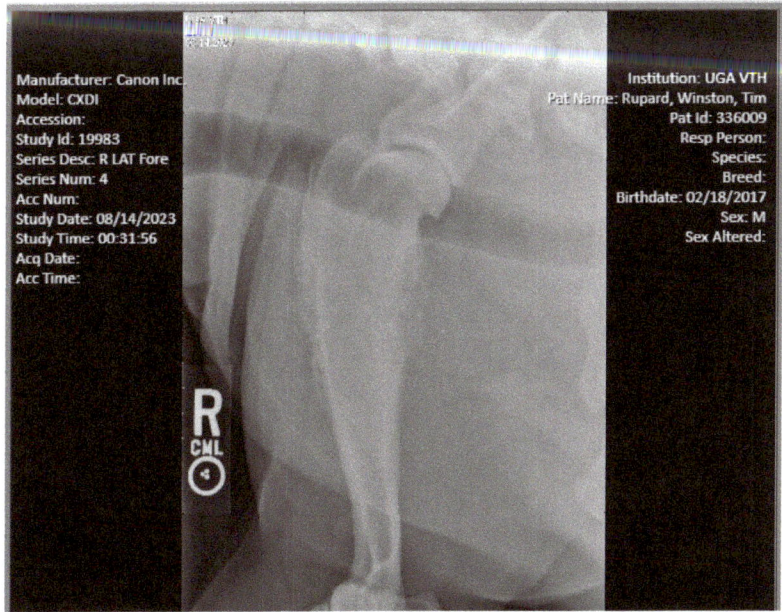

Final xray 8/14/2023 UGA Vetrinarian Medical Center
Showing Periosteal Proliferation

We want, more than anything, to get this book into the hands of everyone who is suffering. If you know anyone who needs a copy, buy one and have it sent. If you cannot buy it, contact us. Also, go here to get a copy of "Winston Wins" the children's book.
Visit our website:
www.winstonstory.com
scan the QR Codes for FB and IG

WEBSITE

INSTAGRAM

FACEBOOK

ACKNOWLEDGEMENTS

SPECIAL THANKS

Before I mention any one person, as I began to jot down the names and reasons I needed to thank the following, I came to the realization that The Father has surrounded me with men and women of God beyond my wildest dreams. Inadequate doesn't begin to describe how I feel when I begin to measure the stature of the Spiritual Giants with whom I am blessed to be among. It is amazing to me to see how each one has had such a specific role and part in all of this. Truly, truly, Karen and I have been blessed, beyond measure, to be held and loved on and encouraged by such great people. We thank you all from the depths of our souls.

To my incredible wife who takes such good notes and journals everything so well. (If she had not, there is no telling how mis-combobulated the chronology of this would be!) I thank her for her patience, for her support, for the hours and hours she spent being a writer's widow as I hacked at the computer, talked over details, discussed the entire project at length with so, so many people. For loving me when I seemed completely insane. For her faith when I was faithless. For her warm compassion when I was broken. For her prayers, she whispered over me, even when I didn't know she was praying. For her direction when I wandered off the path and for her undying love. I love you, Karen, thank you!

To Dewitt for listening to God's voice and going out on a limb that many of us would have shied away from and for being a spiritual encouragement and blessing to us as we have moved forward.

To Heather Webster who spoke into our lives from a vision, God gave her, about the Children's book, WinstonWins (WW), and her willingness to read, edit, suggest, and support us as we chopped our way forward.

To our Pastor, Travis Rutland, for being willing to shepherd us through this time. I have been particularly needy, I believe, as I worked through all of this. He has listened, advised, supported, and written the forward for the book. I cannot express how much we admire and love this man. I love doing ministry with him and learning from him but above all, I value his friendship. Thank you, Pastor.

To my front line warrior friend, John Jennings. I truly wonder if the outcome would have been the same if it had not been for John Jennings. When I remotely faltered in my walking forward through this, John was there, a spiritual drill sergeant, reminding me of who I am and what I am capable of. A source of scriptural reference that boggles the mind, John was there, armed with a word from the Bible to back up whatever it was he was saying. Always ready with a fresh, new word from The Lord about how this was going to go, John wasn't simply "support," John was fuel. John was the catalyst that changed everything about how I believed. I thought I heard God in that vet's office. John removed any doubt and gave me solid ground to stand on about what I thought I heard. I cannot say thank you enough for your willingness to listen to God and do what He says with the passion with which you do it.

To both my parents. Bob and Judy Rupard: For pouring over these works and giving countless suggestions and edits, for Bob's insight and insistence to take Winston to Dalton GA, for my mom's incredible sense of encouragement. These two have always been my biggest fans, and in this endeavor, they have remained true to that statement. To my dear mother who worked tirelessly to make edits and keep my "vernacular" from shining through! She is heaven-sent. Thank you, Mom, for all of your hours, editing and editing again. Thank you both for all you have done.

To my Sister Angela. You have been an incredible source of encouragement and wise counsel. You challenged me to go where I had never gone before and helped me along the way to understand things from perspectives I would never have thought of. You are wise beyond your years and a great friend and sister!

To my loving son, Jonathan Rupard, who has spent nearly as many hours as I did writing, working on the illustrations for both books. For his desire to make sure the images were conveying the truth as much as my every, written word. Jonathan tirelessly poured himself into the drawings with a passion for this project that matched my own. Thank you and God bless you for your talents and willingness to share them.

To my incredible niece, Rebekah Clegg Howard, for her classic photography work for the cover for this book! She always makes things look incredible! Regardless of the time of the morning or year!

To our dear friends Rico and Vikki Ruiz. Rico has calmly steered me through the storm for the last year and a half and is steadfast in his advice and words of encouragement. His spiritual leadership has been beyond imagination through this time.

To Jessica Robinson for perfecting the editing of WW. The one person who has had more experience in reading that type of literature than anyone else involved. She helped me to more clearly communicate on the right level.
To Leslie Rowe for being so willing to help me with water-color painting for WTW. Your knowledge was a true source of grace for me!

To my dear friend Corey Fenn who has walked alongside us through this entire ordeal. Corey was the second person to come to my house and lay his hands on Winston, pray and cry like a baby over his diagnosis and stand with me in faith, believing for the unbelievable. Claiming the power of God over a situation that seemed hopeless. He loaned me his prayer cloth and told me to use it however I felt necessary. He has been a great friend and a huge supporter through the long process. I would not make it without friends like Corey. Update 7/22 Corey is now the proud papa of a puppy from Winston's first litter of offspring. Good luck with all of that buddy!

To Johnny at the Grace bookstore in North, GA. For believing in me, giving me lots of "Bible oil" to pour on Winston and share with others, for your honesty and venerability, for your steadfastness in seeking truth and grace.

To Vickey Bley. If not for you, I may never have found my way to publishing! Thank you so much for your help along the way!

To Katy Chadwick at Brightside Dog Training and Boarding in Dacula, Ga for the gracious use of her facility for some photos for this book and Winston Wins. www.brightsidedogtraining.com

To Dr. Jeremy Adams. (Adams Chiropractic Clinic) For your continued faith and support and for bending all the rules to X-ray my dog in your facility! Be Blessed My friend!

To Nancy LaPier for putting in the extra hours for a final edit before going to my latest print. It just wouldn't read as well without your expertise and hard work! Thank you so much, Nancy!

Most of all, to Jesus Christ, who was beaten for our sickness, bore our sins on the cross and rose again on the 3rd day to defeat sickness and death in our place. Who led me to this moment in my life, through the Holy Spirit, to share this portion of our lives with you.

BIO
TIM A RUPARD

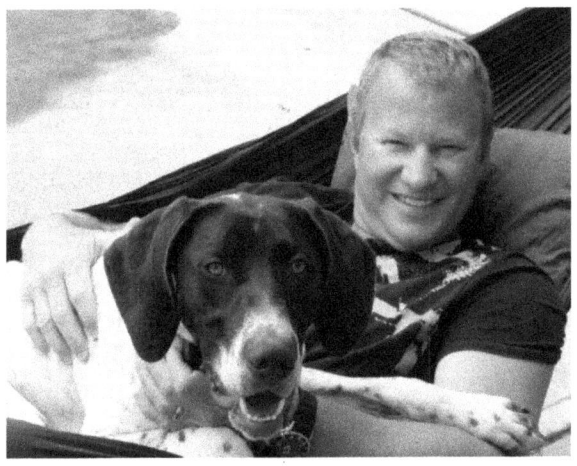

Tim and Heidi

Tim has been described as a craftsman on many levels. However, he most enjoys the craft of story-telling. He writes often, as an outlet for expression, although he doesn't formally consider himself a "writer." He has written a few published articles for a news paper in a nearby city, and has a blog for his personal website to which he contributes quarterly.

Tim owns his own business and works at his church as the missions pastor and the men's pastor. He is a husband to an incredible woman, Karen, a father, step father and father-in-law to six incredible people. Jon and Kat, Ashley, Kaitlyn and Kevin and Abby. He is also a grandfather to arguably the three best little boys and the two most beautiful and best little girls in the world.

He is an avid outdoors-man and typically prefers to be outside over in. It is his love of the outdoors that drives many of his habits, character traits, and stories. He believes God speaks to him often through his time spent out-of-doors and hopes to relay those moments as effectively as possible, in his writings.

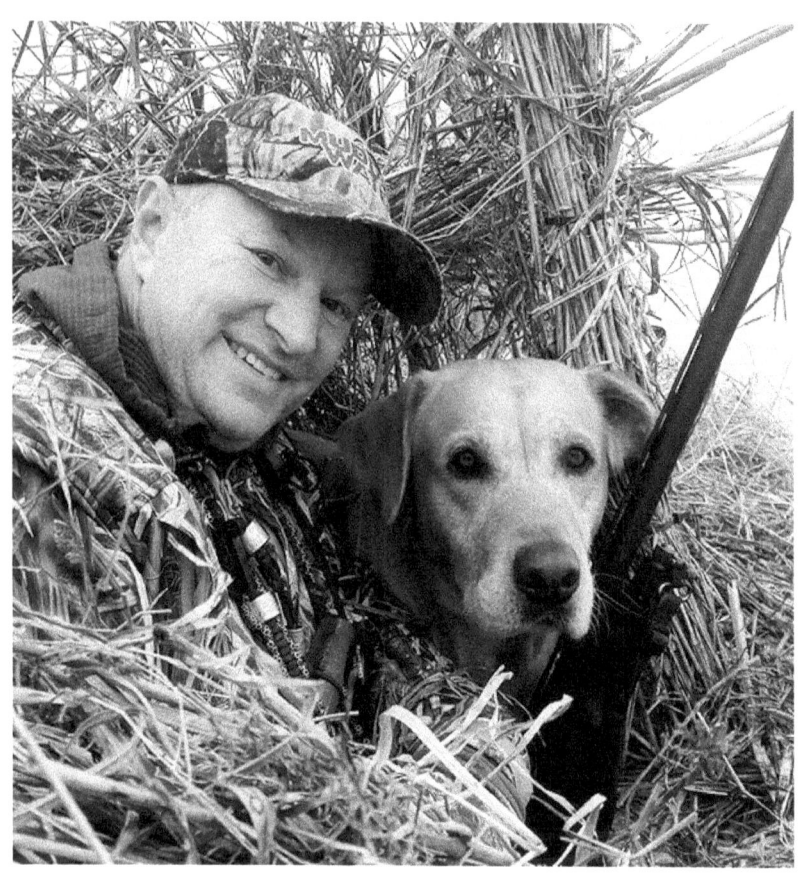

Tim and Winston in the winter duck season of 2020. After Winston was healed of cancer, he has resumed the normal life of a working Lab.
Well, almost normal.

APPENDIX

1 Death rate per accident https://apnews.com/b54947eac455d4ec896ae126d0f86eac

2 The deadliest cars of all time
https://www.thrillist.com/cars/the-deadliest-vehicles-of-all-time-iihs-driver-death-rates-and-mercedes-at-lemans

3 Sermon From Travis Rutland, "Sensing Jesus" 11/14/21

4 Quote from Curry Blake Series DHT Training, Youtube.